SURGEON'S KNIFE
Head and Neck Incisions

SURGEON'S KNIFE
Head and Neck Incisions

Mohammad Akheel
BDS MDS FHNCS FADI FIIHNO
Associate Head and Neck Oncosurgeon
Department of Surgical Oncology
The Convenient Hospital Ltd. (CHL)–
Comprehensive Blood and Cancer Center (CBCC)
Visiting Consultant, Global SNG Hospitals
and Shalby Hospitals
Indore, Madhya Pradesh, India

Co-author
Ashmi Wadhwania
BDS MDS PGDEMS
Consultant Oral and Maxillofacial Surgeon
Modern Dental Care
Surat, Gujarat, India

Forewords
Jatin P Shah
Iype Cherian
Mayte Pinilla Urraca

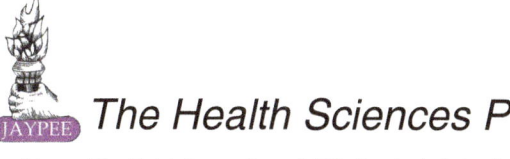

The Health Sciences Publisher
New Delhi | London | Philadelphia | Panama

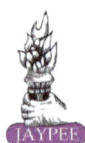 **Jaypee Brothers Medical Publishers (P) Ltd**

Headquarters

Jaypee Brothers Medical Publishers (P) Ltd
4838/24, Ansari Road, Daryaganj
New Delhi 110 002, India
Phone: +91-11-43574357
Fax: +91-11-43574314
Email: jaypee@jaypeebrothers.com

Overseas Offices

J.P. Medical Ltd
83 Victoria Street, London
SW1H 0HW (UK)
Phone: +44 20 3170 8910
Fax: +44 (0)20 3008 6180
Email: info@jpmedpub.com

Jaypee Medical Inc
325 Chestnut Street
Suite 412, Philadelphia, PA 19106, USA
Phone: +1 267-519-9789
Email: support@jpmedus.com

Jaypee Brothers Medical Publishers (P) Ltd
Bhotahity, Kathmandu
Nepal
Phone: +977-9741283608
Email: kathmandu@jaypeebrothers.com

Jaypee-Highlights Medical Publishers Inc
City of Knowledge, Bld. 235, 2nd Floor, Clayton
Panama City, Panama
Phone: +1 507-301-0496
Fax: +1 507-301-0499
Email: cservice@jphmedical.com

Jaypee Brothers Medical Publishers (P) Ltd
17/1-B Babar Road, Block-B, Shaymali
Mohammadpur, Dhaka-1207
Bangladesh
Mobile: +08801912003485
Email: jaypeedhaka@gmail.com

Website: www.jaypeebrothers.com
Website: www.jaypeedigital.com

© 2016, Jaypee Brothers Medical Publishers

The views and opinions expressed in this book are solely those of the original contributor(s)/author(s) and do not necessarily represent those of editor(s) of the book.

All rights reserved. No part of this publication may be reproduced, stored or transmitted in any form or by any means, electronic, mechanical, photocopying, recording or otherwise, without the prior permission in writing of the publishers.

All brand names and product names used in this book are trade names, service marks, trademarks or registered trademarks of their respective owners. The publisher is not associated with any product or vendor mentioned in this book.

Medical knowledge and practice change constantly. This book is designed to provide accurate, authoritative information about the subject matter in question. However, readers are advised to check the most current information available on procedures included and check information from the manufacturer of each product to be administered, to verify the recommended dose, formula, method and duration of administration, adverse effects and contraindications. It is the responsibility of the practitioner to take all appropriate safety precautions. Neither the publisher nor the author(s)/editor(s) assume any liability for any injury and/or damage to persons or property arising from or related to use of material in this book.

This book is sold on the understanding that the publisher is not engaged in providing professional medical services. If such advice or services are required, the services of a competent medical professional should be sought.

Every effort has been made where necessary to contact holders of copyright to obtain permission to reproduce copyright material. If any have been inadvertently overlooked, the publisher will be pleased to make the necessary arrangements at the first opportunity.

Inquiries for bulk sales may be solicited at: jaypee@jaypeebrothers.com

SURGEON'S KNIFE Head and Neck Incisions

First Edition: **2016**

ISBN: 978-93-86056-86-3

Dedicated to

Almighty Allah
My Parents and Family
My Life Partner
My Teachers
and
My Friends

Foreword

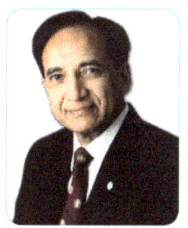

"Look before you leap" and "Think before you act" are the aphorisms that come into play, every time a surgeon takes a scalpel in his hand. A poorly planned and ill-placed incision, may not only be a frustrating exercise for the surgeon due to inadequate exposure but may also lead to lifelong unhappiness on the part of the patient with poor aesthetic outcome and often significant functional compromise. An ideal incision is one which offers the surgeon the required operative exposure to do an optimal operative procedure without compromise and leaves the patient with minimal aesthetic impact and little if any functional loss.

In order for the surgeon to choose the ideal incision, knowledge of neurovascular anatomy of the skin and underlying muscles, patient's body habitus, and respect to natural skin creases and Langer's lines is essential. In addition, in planning the incision, the possibility of extension of the incision to embark upon unanticipated additional or more extensive operative procedures must be taken into account. The need for future surgery must be kept in mind, such as the possibility of a neck dissection after an open biopsy of a neck node, where the biopsy incision should be able to be incorporated in the eventual incision for neck dissection.

Dr Mohammad Akheel is to be congratulated for putting together an outstanding compendium on the incisions, both old and new, applicable in various procedures in the head and neck region. This comprehensive treatise of a large variety of incisions employed by surgeons of the past era and present times offers the reader a menu of the surgical approaches for congenital conditions, trauma and tumor surgery as well as reconstructive surgery.

The surgeon has an opportunity to select the appropriate incision to employ in a given setting from this large list of approaches described, keeping in mind the pros and cons of each incision for the procedure at hand. This book would be of great value to the students and trainees of maxillofacial surgery, dental surgery, otolaryngology, general surgery, head and neck surgery and plastic surgery.

It would also be a tremendous resource in the libraries of dental and medical schools, as well as clinical departments where surgery in the head and neck region is being practiced.

Jatin P Shah, MD, PhD(Hon), DSc(Hon),
FACS FRCS (Hon) FDSRCS (Hon) FRCSDS (Hon) FRACS (Hon)
E W Strong Chair in Head and Neck Oncology
Memorial Sloan Kettering Cancer Center
New York, USA

Foreword

It has been an honor knowing Dr Akheel. He has the passion to excel and has been on the constant mode of never-ending improvement. It is heartening to see him run up the stairs of success. With this book, he has completed another milestone. The book is easy to read and informative and has been presented in a very interesting way. I am sure the target audience of skull base surgeons and maxillofacial surgeons would benefit a lot. I wish Dr Akheel all the best in the near future and would be waiting to see him go further.

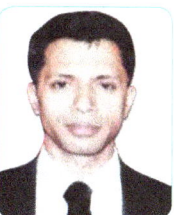

Iype Cherian, MCh Neurosurgery (CMC, Vellore)
Professor and Head, Department of Neurosurgery
College of Medical Sciences, Bharatpur, Chitwan, Nepal
Counselor General-Asian Congress of Neurological Surgeons
Incharge, ACNS Education Courses
International EB Member, Surgical Neurology International
AJNS Chief Editor, ACNS Surgical Manual
Faculty, WFNS Anatomy Committee

Foreword

It is a pleasure to read and to recommend this interesting book by Dr Mohammad Akheel. Since I met him, he has not done anything but surprising me with his scientific interest and attempt to improve surgical medical knowledge of his specialty. This book is a summary of all facial and skull incisions from the oldest to the most current as well as the flaps for reconstruction of defects created after the surgery of this area. It is a book of great interest not only to medical 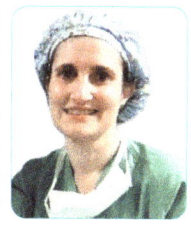 residents but also to medical specialists with interest in head and neck surgery as maxillofacial, plastic and ENT to give a clear, brief and iconographic way to perform these surgical approaches.

Mayte Pinilla Urraca, MD PhD
Deputy Chief, Department of Otolaryngology
Hospital Universitario Puerta de Hierro Majadahonda
Madrid, Spain

Preface

FACE IS THE INDEX OF OUR MIND!!!

This is an old saying which says face is a part of body which helps us to convey our thinking, feelings and other emotions. A knife is like a sword in surgeon's hand which gives life to his patients. This book is an atlas which covers all incisions of head and neck region providing a valuable piece of information for residents/specialists practising head and neck surgery. I hope the readers will have the feeling of rapture after reading this book.

I have tried to cover all the incisions of particular region starting from the historical ones and till date with references. The understanding of the face as a compact dynamic emotional structure has been changed more during the last 30 years than during the last 20,000 years. The surgeon's task is not only to incise the facial structures but also to rejuvenate it, and also to harmonize, enhance and symmetrize it. In order to achieve this, the very first step of placing a knife to make an incision needs a meticulous planning. This book shall help the young surgeon/resident to know about various incisions, practice a safe and ethical surgery to avoid inadvertent complications. Planning an incision in the facial region is an art and needs a proper knowledge about facial architecture. A wrong incision can make you land in legal problems.

Hence, this book will help you to know all the incisions under one roof, and I hope there is no book other than by Sir Edward Ellis III which summarizes all these incisions together. I wish you good luck in all your future endeavors and enjoy reading this atlas.

Mohammad Akheel

Acknowledgments

I am very thankful to Almighty Allah for instilling the idea of writing of this book and helping me in all my endeavors.

I am very thankful and obliged to my father, Mohammad Hameed, my mother Tahera Sultana and my brother Mohammad Afroz who are always there as my support, and whatever I am today is due to their prayers, love and affection.

I am very thankful to my Co-author, my inspiration and my beloved life partner Dr Ashmi Wadhwania, a gorgeous maxillofacial surgeon with beauty and brain, without whose help and contribution this book might have not been possible.

I sincerely thank my fellowship guides Dr Raj Nagarkar (Chairman and Surgical Oncologist) and Dr Sirshendu Roy (Surgical Oncologist) of HCG Curie Manavata Cancer Center, Nashik, Maharashtra, for giving me an opportunity to learn oncology and thereby making my dream to come true.

I sincerely thank my postgraduate and undergraduate teachers who have taught me that academics and discipline are two important things in life which makes a man successful in his career.

I thank my mentor, my guide and my friend Dr Suryapratap Singh Tomar, a young and dynamic neuro and spine surgeon from India who has shaped me and made me realize my potential.

I am sincerely thankful to Dr Niyaz Wadhwania, a third year student of Bachelor of Dental Surgery (BDS), MA Rangoonwala Dental College, Pune, Maharashtra, who has volunteered for the photographs of incisions for this book.

In the end, I would like to thank all my friends who have always motivated me in all my academic works.

Author's View

FACE—A DYNAMIC MOSAIC WORK

The aesthetic expectations of an increasingly young population have changed considerably over the last 10 years. Not only the young but also the aging population has a different view about the facial aesthetics which was neglected some years back. Our senior plastic surgeons are developing more newer techniques to give a maximum aesthetic appeal to the face.

According to me, the face is now considered as 3-dimensional dynamic mosaic work. Numerous techniques are now available to improve the arrangement of these facial pieces in the mosaic. Now we can achieve more sustainable harmonic results while reducing the potential risks and complications to get a good harmony when performing any elective facial procedure. It is of utmost importance that the surgeon listens carefully to his/her patient's wishes and expectations. Hence, in this way, we can make a plan for the placement of our incision mostly in the inconspicuous area of head and neck and also the length of incision to have an adequate exposure of area to be operated. Any artificial/iatrogenic mark on the face of the patient will lower their social self-esteem. Hence, a surgeon must keep this in mind and rejuvenate the face near to the original architecture to satisfy the patient's social and psychological appeal.

Here, again I stress on this point that the biggest risk in any type of head and neck surgery lies in the surgeon himself/herself. If he/she has not received excellent education and exposure of the various types of incisions/approaches to the facial structures, if he/she lacks sufficient experience, then the patient is exposed to an enormous risk of facial disharmony. There is also a global phenomenon that surgically untrained physicians and even nonphysicians, maxillofacial surgeons, and cosmeticians are offering aesthetic surgeries. Aesthetic or cosmetic surgery is enjoying ever-increasing popularity and social acceptance but only when it is done by appropriate planning. Hence, my humble request to all the budding head and neck surgeons—PLAN YOUR INCISION EVEN BEFORE YOU HAVE A KNIFE IN YOUR HAND!!!

Mohammad Akheel

Contents

1. Fourth Dimension of Face — 1
2. Principles of Incision — 2
3. Concepts of Incision — 6
4. Principles of Reconstruction — 9
5. Third Molar Impactions — 10
6. Maxillofacial Fractures — 13
7. Space Infections — 24
8. Neoplasms — 26
9. Cleft Lip — 44
10. Cleft Palate — 49
11. Temporomandibular Joint — 51
12. Flaps — 60
13. Aesthetic Surgery — 74

Bibliography — *79*
Index — *81*

CHAPTER 1

Fourth Dimension of Face

The most important surface full of secrets which we face is the "FACE". It is curved, sometimes smooth or rough and has its anatomical depth of muscles, nerves, vessels, fat tissues, and ligaments. *But it also has a fourth dimension—that is its spiritual deepness reflecting our mind and soul.*

Face is the tool expressing our emotions, thoughts and messages of surprisingly deep contents in endless floating nuances. We use our face for activities like breathing, eating, drinking, speaking, and hearing. Four senses are concentrated here even the fifth sense called the tactile sense is represented here in face. A single look at the face can make us recognize someone's gender, age, health, race, even affection and individuality. It possesses unique anatomy which has expressiveness, beauty, and singularity. There are more than 10 billion faces on earth and no two of the faces are similar. Even mono-ovular twins have symmetry of their faces, composed like in a mirror but not 100% same in mosaic architecture. We have learned more about the face in the last 30 years than in the 20,000 years before. Every human being has a unique and unmistakable iris, pattern of the ears, and thermic emission of the face and, in addition, the voice, fingerprints, and handwriting are unique. If we imagine that facial muscles are musicians in an orchestra, then the game of our facial expressions would be the melody played by this orchestra. The expressive messages of our faces are universally equally produced and understood—we may speak of facial Esperanto.

CHAPTER

2

Principles of Incision

"KNOW YOUR ANATOMY BEFORE YOU PLACE AN INCISION"

INTRODUCTION

The surgery is often successful when the area to be operated is exposed enough for the surgeon's visibility, accessibility and his instrumentation. As mentioned in Ellis textbook, in orthopedic surgery, especially of the long bone fractures, the basic rule is to have a direct approach to fix the underlying fracture. Therefore, irrespective of important and vital structures, incisions are often placed on or near the fracture site and this involves minimal or no aesthetic concerns.

Head and neck surgical incisions differ from those orthopedic incisions with major concern being the facial aesthetics. Often the incision is placed away from the operated site in the inconspicuous area of the head and neck which can provide enough access and exposure to the operating surgeon. Placing an incision in conspicuous area can create a facial deformity and disharmony which can in turn create a low social self-esteem. In the era of 21st century, aesthetics is the prime importance and a demand of every patient, doesn't matter how severe is the problem. In this atlas, all the incisions are portrayed which are placed in inconspicuous areas of face. To know the planning of incision, one must be thorough of head and neck muscles, most importantly muscles of facial expression.

While placing the incision in head and neck region, one must be careful about its underlying important vital structures. Most important is Cranial Nerve VII (facial nerve). Damage to any of the branches of facial nerve supplying its muscle of facial expression can paralyze the face causing severe facial disharmony.

What is a scalpel or a knife?

Surgical scalpel is like a blade which consists of two parts: a blade and a handle. In these, the handles are reusable (autoclavable) while blades are used only once even when for a small cuts. Hence, they have to be replaced after single use. The handle is also known as "B.P." handle. It is named after Sir Charles Russell Bard and Sir Morgan Parker, founders of the Bard-Parker Company.

The handle of medical scalpels come in two basic types. The first is a flat handle used in the #3 and #4 handles. The #7 handle is more like a long writing pen, rounded at the front and flat at the back. A #4 handle is larger than #3. Blades are manufactured with a corresponding filament size so that they fit on only one size handle.

Surgical Blades

Different types of surgical scalpel blades are discussed in Table 1.

TABLE 1: Types of surgical scalpel blades

Blade No.	Compatible Handles	Blade Description	Uses
No. 10	B3, 3, 3 Graduated, 3 Long, 5, 7, 9	Curved cutting edge with an unsharpened back edge. A more traditional blade shape	Generally for making incisions in skin and muscle. Commonly used to cut the skin in abdominal operations
No. 11	B3, 3, 3 Graduated, 3 Long, 5, 7, 9	Triangular blade with sharp point, flat cutting edge parallel to the handle and flat back	For precision cutting, stripping, sharp angle cuts and also stencil cutting due to its similarity to the X-Acto art knife blade
No. 15	B3, 3, 3 Graduated, 3 Long, 5, 7, 9	A smaller version of the #10	For the same general use as the #10 blade
No. 15C	B3, 3, 3 Graduated, 3 Long, 5, 7, 9	The #15 with a downward angle, flatter and thinner than the #15	The downward angle makes this the preferred blade for working within the chest during cardiac surgery, and is commonly used to make the distal arteriotomy during coronary artery bypass grafting
No. 16	B3, 3, 3 Graduated, 3 Long, 5, 7, 9	A narrow chisel-like blade with flat, angled cutting edge, positioned higher than the axis of the handle	For cutting stencils, scoring and etching
No. 17	B3, 3, 3 Graduated, 3 Long, 5, 7, 9	A flat face 1.6 mm chisel blade	For narrow cuts
No. 18	4, 4 Graduated, 4 Long, 6	A 12.7 mm chisel blade	For deep cuts and scraping
No. 20	4, 4 Graduated, 4 Long, 6	A larger version of the #10 blade, with a curved cutting edge and a flat, unsharpened back edge	Used in general surgery and orthopedic surgery

Contd...

Contd...

No. 22	2, 4, 5, 6	A slightly larger version of the #20, with a curved cutting edge and a flat, unsharpened back edge	Used for skin incisions in both cardiac and thoracic surgery, and to cut the bronchus in lung resection surgery
No. 23	4, 4 Graduated, 4 Long, 6	Similar to #22, leaf-shaped	For long incisions
No. 24	4, 4 Graduated, 4 Long, 6	A wide, flat, angled cutting edge	For corner cuts, trimming, stripping, and cutting mats and gaskets
No. 36	4, 4 Graduated, 4 Long, 6	A larger blade	Used in general surgery but also within a Laboratory setting for Histology and Histopathology

Basic principles

Following factors are important when the incision is being planned. They are patient's gender, age, amount of lax skin, anatomical disturbances and his/her expectations. The age of the patient is important because of the presence of wrinkles and lax skin which can hide the incision in natural skin lines. Existing anatomic features that are unique to the individual can also facilitate or hamper incision placement. For example, any preexisting scar can hamper the placement of fresh incision. In most of the cases, this scar can be used to expose the underlying skeleton or area to be operated. Patient's expectations and wishes must always be considered in any decision about location of an incision.

Principles of Placing an Incision

The following steps are important to place an incision:
1. Incisions are placed by holding the knife at 45°–50° to the skin.
2. Incisions are placed in inconspicuous area of face.
3. If given an option of extraoral or intraoral incision, preference should be given to intraoral incision.
4. Avoid important neurovascular structures when you place an incision.
5. The length of the incision must be restricted to provide enough working space for accessibility, visibility and instrumentation.
6. The depth of the incision must be till subdermal layer.
7. Place the incision perpendicular to the surface of nonhair bearing skin. Incisions placed obliquely to the surface of skin are susceptible for marginal necrosis.
8. Place the incision in the lines of minimal tension also called as relaxed skin tension lines. These lines are skin's adaptation to function and the elastic nature to the underlying dermis. The chronic contractions of the muscles

create deep creases. These lines are good choice to place an incision and the resulting scar is hidden.
9. If incisions cannot be placed in inconspicuous areas, get help from local anatomical structures. For example, place the incision intraorally, nose, ear, eyelid or inside the hair bearing area.
10. Closure of incisions of surgical sites must be in layers to prevent contracture of tissues.

CHAPTER

3

Concepts of Incision

Obtaining accurate knowledge and assessment of nearby soft tissues and skeletal structures is crucial before making an incision.

The face consists of six major aesthetic units comprised of forehead, eye/eyebrow, nose, lips, chin, and cheek. These aesthetic units can be subdivided into additional anatomical subunits. For example, the nose can be divided into nasal tip, dorsum, columella, soft tissue triangles, sidewalls, and nasal alar regions.

Facial aesthetic units and subunits are visual anatomical boundaries. Light reflections and shadows along these facial aesthetic borders help conceal parallel scars. Evaluate skin laxity surrounding the planned incision. Appreciate the key functional and aesthetic structures nearby, such as cranial nerves and mobile facial structures (e.g. eyelids, nasal alae, nasal tip, auricle, vermilion, commissures, philtral ridges).

Correct orientation of planned incisions next to these mobile functional and aesthetic facial structures is important to avoid distortion when closing wounds. Optimally, perform an incision or an excision within or parallel to the relaxed skin-tension lines (RSTLs) of the face (Fig. 1).

The image shows relaxed skin-tension lines (RSTLs) of the face as seen on magnified facial image. Examples of drawn optimal fusiform excisions run parallel to RSTLs. Specifically, RSTLs can be defined as the skin-tension lines that are oriented along the furrows formed when skin is relaxed. The resting tone and contractile forces of underlying facial musculature perpendicular to skin-tension lines contribute to RSTLs. Unlike wrinkle lines, RSTLs are not clearly visible on the skin. While pinching the skin, however, RSTLs can be observed from the furrows and ridges thus revealed.

The closer an incision comes to lying within an RSTL, the better the ultimate cosmetic appearance of the scar. If possible, avoid making incisions perpendicular to RSTLs because the greatest amount of lax skin lies perpendicular to RSTLs.

In addition to planning incisions along RSTLs or at the border of facial aesthetic units (i.e. forehead, eye/eyebrow, nose, lips, chin, cheek), adherence

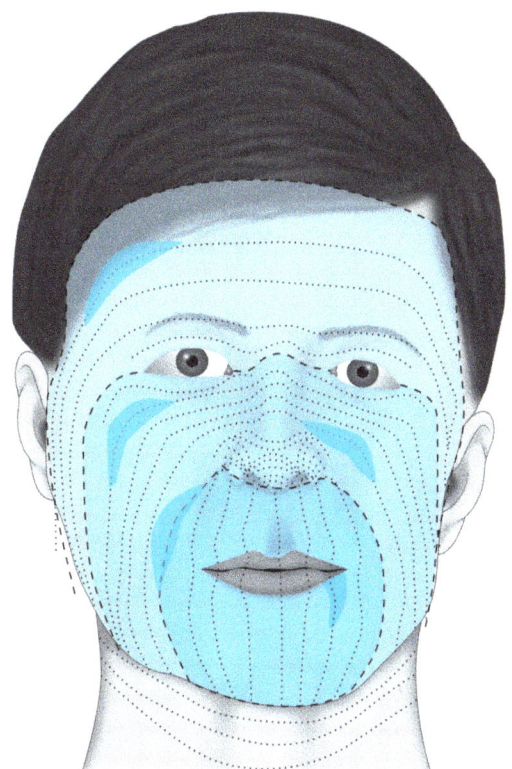

Fig. 1: Relaxed skin-tension lines of the face as seen on magnified facial image

to techniques of tensionless wound closure, wound edge eversion, and atraumatic handling of tissues optimizes scar appearance. Preoperatively marking the sitting patient with a surgical pen helps determine the effect of gravity on the surrounding tissue around the planned incision. Furthermore, it helps give a more accurate assessment of the planned incision in respect to the relaxed skin-tension lines before local anesthesia is injected.

In elective facial cosmetic surgery, proper preoperative incision planning is crucial. This is because one of the major priorities of cosmetic facial surgery is to maximally conceal surgical incisions. For example, in facelift surgery, the telltale signs of poorly placed incisions are temporal hair loss, unnatural appearance of the ear tragus, and posterior hairline distortion. In addition, for the male patient, special consideration is given by modifying facelift incisions in the preauricular area.

In reconstructive head and neck surgery, proper planning of neck incisions are important to prevent carotid artery exposure if skin breakdown should occur after a radical neck dissection. If a wound cannot be closed primarily, reconstructive options may include using skin flaps or grafts for which the design of the incisions follows the same aesthetic unit and RSTL principles.

Reconstructive options include healing by secondary intention, local or regional flaps, or skin grafts. When removal of the majority of a facial aesthetic unit is anticipated, excision of the remaining aesthetic skin unit can be considered before reconstructive coverage. This can help minimize scars by having them lie along the aesthetic unit boundaries. When a defect encompasses more than one aesthetic unit, each unit can be reconstructed as a separate entity.

When considering incisions for local flap coverage, take advantage of the cutaneous vascular regions of the face to optimize viability of the flap and insure primary healing. These vascular regions are defined by the four main paired arteries of the face, which majorly provide blood supply to facial skin. Major arteries to the facial skin are (1) the supratrochlear artery, which contributes to the central forehead and palpebral region; (2) the supraorbital artery, which perfuses the medial forehead region; (3) the temporal artery, which branches into superficial temporal and transverse facial arteries supplying the temporal forehead, lateral cheek, and periauricular regions; and (4) the facial artery, which leads into the superior and inferior labial, angular, and palpebral arteries, thereby perfusing the central and lower midface.

In planning elective procedures, over-the-counter products that decrease clotting should be discontinued, if possible, 14 days before incisions are made. These products include aspirin, aspirin-related products, gingko biloba, ginseng, flax seed, and vitamin E. This is because a decreased ability to clot increases the risk for hematoma formation and later subdermal fibrosis, resulting in skin elevation (pincushioning).

CHAPTER

4

Principles of Reconstruction

There are certain principles for reconstructing the hard and soft tissue defects which has to be followed by every reconstructive surgeon. Most of the time, reconstruction is done by resection team of surgeons. In these cases, the ideal principles of reconstruction might be unknowingly violated. Hence, there is a need to have a separate reconstruction team.

Gillie's Principles of Reconstruction

The following are some principles given by Gillie's and Milliard.
1. **First, fully diagnose the problem before trying to treat it. Then make a plan**—Before starting any treatment, have a good clinical diagnosis of the problem with all the adjuvant investigations required and then make a plan.
2. **Make a plan, a pattern of the plan, and have a lifeboat**—Make a plan with all steps. Try to have a plan B, if plan A fails to save yourself.
3. **Treat the primary defect first**—Treat the problem first.
4. **Not to discard anything**—Do not discard any soft or hard tissues. Try to save as much as possible.
5. **Returning tissues to their normal position**—Try to return the tissues back to the normal position to maintain the facial architecture and harmony.
6. **Replacing lost tissue by similar tissue**—Try to replace the lost tissue with more or less similar kind of tissue from some other area which matches its color and consistency.
7. **Not to do today what can honorably be put off till tomorrow (when in doubt, don't)**—When in doubt, don't be in hurry to reconstruct the primary defect. If you suspect of recurrence/irradiated tissue then wait for 3-6 months and then plan for reconstruction.
8. **Treat each case individually**—Each case is different. Do not interrelate with other case. Plan according to the case strictly.
Millard (1995)—We must maintain superiority in our special three P's—**philosophy, principles, and perfection** of execution.

CHAPTER
5

Third Molar Impactions

Flap design is important, not only for allowing optimal visibility and access to the impacted tooth, but also for subsequent healing of the surgically created defect. There are various incisions for third molar impactions.

Ward's Incision (Fig. 1)

Ward's incision consists of three limb. Anterior limb starts from distobuccal line angle of second molar extending obliquely downwards. It is usually half an inch. Intermediate limb is usually a crevicular incision. Posterior or distal limb starts from the most posterior teeth to the external oblique ridge.

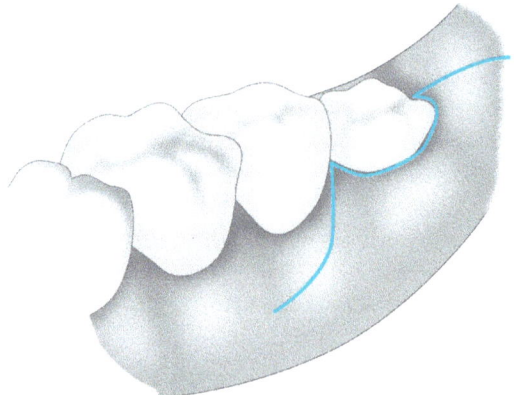

Fig. 1: Ward's incision

Modified Ward's Incision (Fig. 2)

Modified ward's incision consists of three limbs. Anterior limb starts from distobuccal line angle to first molar extending obliquely downwards. It is usually half an inch. Intermediate limb is usually a crevicular incision. Posterior or distal limb starts from the most posterior teeth to the external oblique ridge.

Third Molar Impactions

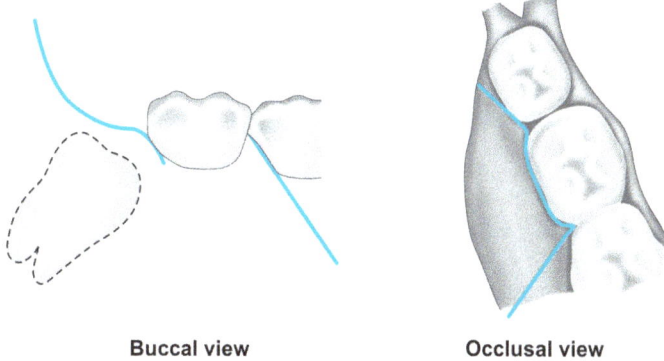

Buccal view **Occlusal view**

Fig. 2: Modified ward's incision

L-shaped Incision (Fig. 3)

Usually used for completely impacted tooth. It has two limbs. Anterior or vertical limb starts from distal to second molar and posterior limb along the crest running along the ascending border of ramus.

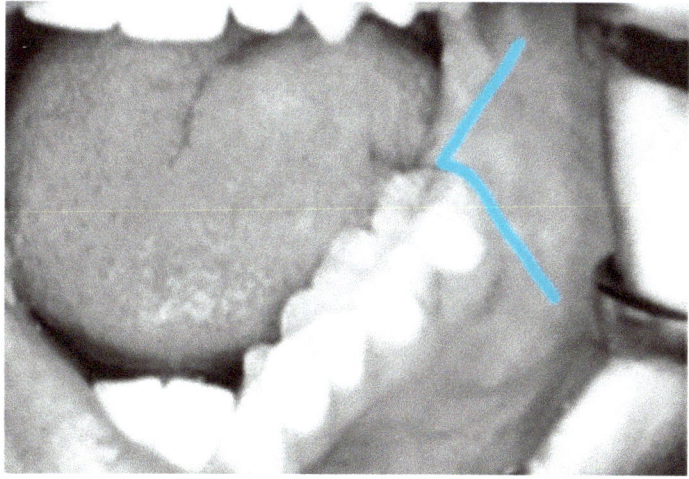

Fig. 3: L-shaped incision

Comma Incision (Fig. 4)

Comma incision was given by Nageshwar in 2002. It is a minimal invasive incision starting from a point which is at the depth of stretched vestibular reflection which is posterior to the distal aspect of the preceding second molar, the incision is made in an anterior direction. Incision is made to a point below the second molar, from where it is smoothly curved up to meet the gingival crest at the distobuccal line angle of the second molar. The incision is continued as a crevicular incision around the distal aspect of the second molar.

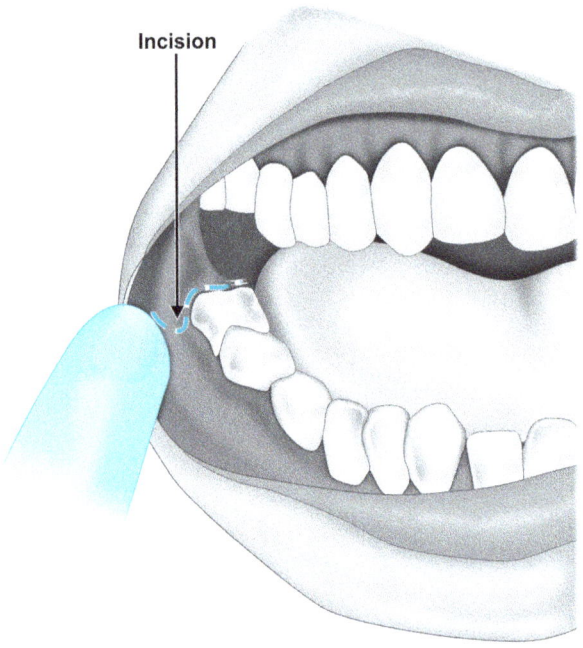

Fig. 4: Comma incision

Envelope Incision (Fig. 5)

Envelope incision is a crevicular type of incision. It may or may not have a distal limb.

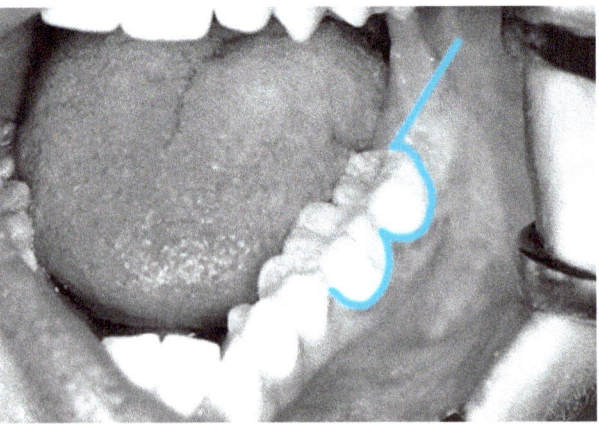

Fig. 5: Envelope incision

CHAPTER

6

Maxillofacial Fractures

This chapter is divided into many subdivisions which will cover all the extraoral and intraoral incisions to approach the fracture line.

MANDIBULAR FRACTURES

Extraoral Incisions

Submandibular (Risdon's) Approach

The initial incision, which is about 3.0 cm long, is made through the skin and subcutaneous tissues to the level of the platysma muscle. It is placed either 1.0 or 2.0 cm below and parallel to the lower border of the mandible or slightly lower so that it is located in or parallel to a skin crease. The lower location generally produces a less conspicuous scar.

The main structures to be avoided are the marginal mandibular branch of the facial nerve and the retromandibular vein. The marginal mandibular branch of the facial nerve, posterior to the facial artery, pass above the inferior border of the mandible in 81% of dissections **(Dingman, Grabb, 1962)**. It runs superficial to the facial vein in all the cadavers studied. It can, however, run as much as 3 cm below the inferior border of the mandible, deep to the platysma muscle. The dissection is carried down through skin, subcutaneous tissue, and platysma. A nerve stimulator is used to identify the mandibular branch, and it is retracted superiorly.

This incision is used for fractures of body and angle of mandible (Fig. 1).
- First Incision—Incision parallel to lower border of mandible
- Second Incision—Incision in neck crease.

Retromandibular Incision

A 3.0–3.5 cm incision is made through the skin and subcutaneous tissues just posterior and parallel to the posterior border of the ascending ramus, extending from a point just below the level of the lobule of the ear inferiorly to a point just above the angle of the mandible (Fig. 2).

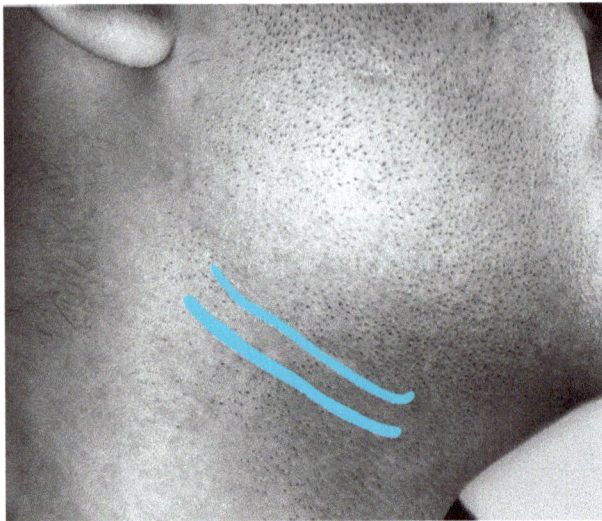

Fig. 1: Submandibular approach

This incision is used for angle of the mandible, ramus of the mandible and condyle of the mandible.

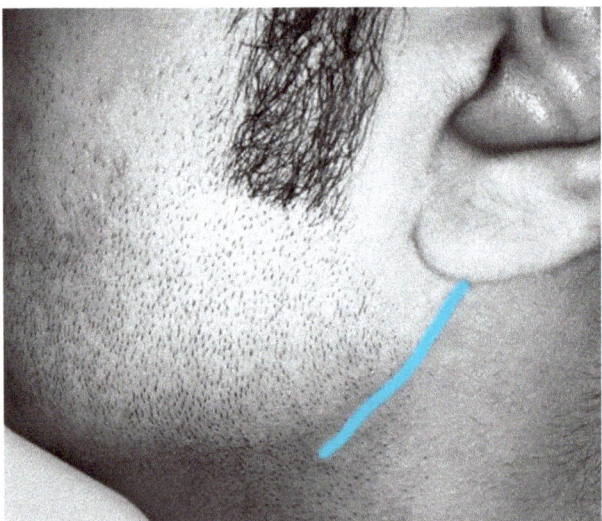

Fig. 2: Retromandibular incision

Intraoral Incisions (Figs 3A and B)

Vestibular Incisions

This is an intraoral incision placed in vestibular sulcus for fractures of symphysis, parasymphysis, body and angle. This provides better cosmesis than other extraoral incisions.

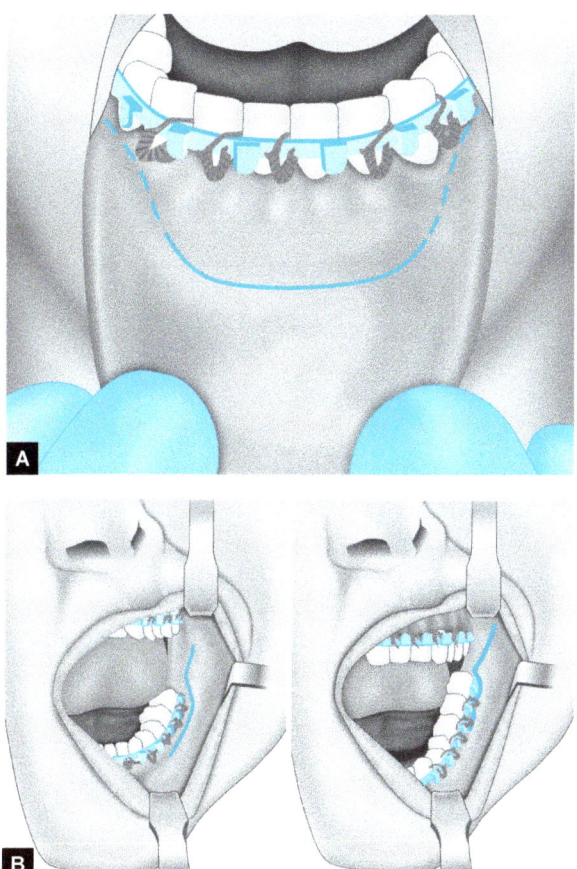

Figs 3A and B: Intraoral incisions—Vestibular incisions

MAXILLARY FRACTURES

Vestibular Incision (Fig. 4)

Fractures of anterior wall of maxilla can be approached by **Midfacial degloving approach.**

ZYGOMATIC COMPLEX FRACTURES

Extraoral Incisions

Lateral brow incision: An approximately 2 cm long horizontal incision is marked within the bounds of the lateral eyebrow parallel to hair follicles (Fig. 5).

Infraorbital incision: The lower-eyelid incision is ideal for exposing the orbital floor, the orbital rim, and the lateral orbital wall (Fig. 6).

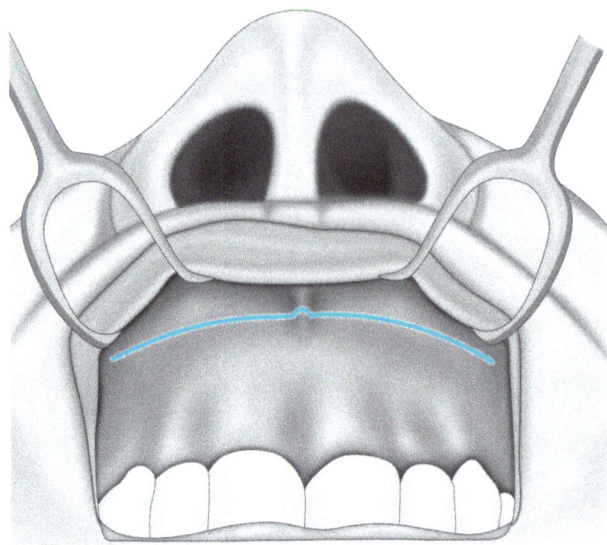

Fig. 4: Maxillary fractures—vestibular incision

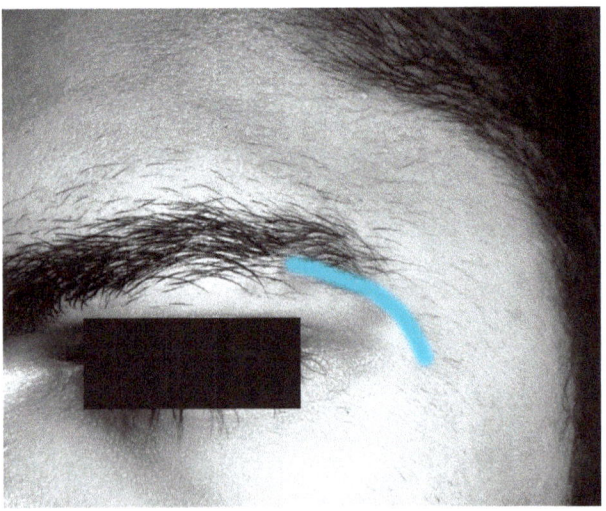

Fig. 5: Lateral brow incisions

Gillie's approach: Incision given between the two branches of superficial temporal artery (Fig. 7).

Percutaneous approach: Stab incision given in meeting point of imaginary line drawn from tragus to ala of nose and line dropped from lateral canthus of eye.

Maxillofacial Fractures | 17

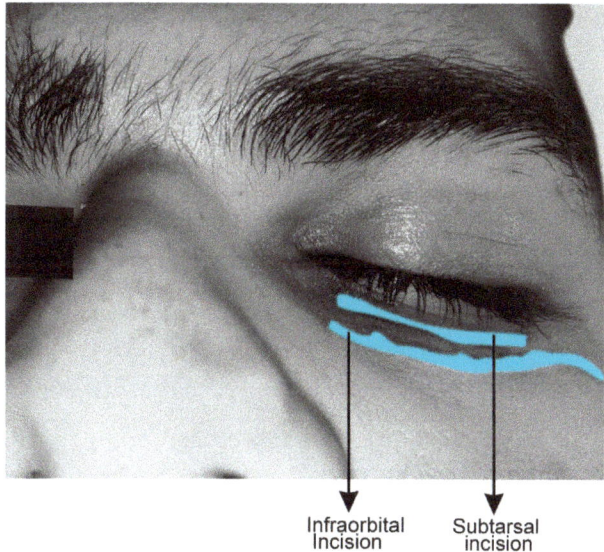

Fig. 6: Infraorbital incision

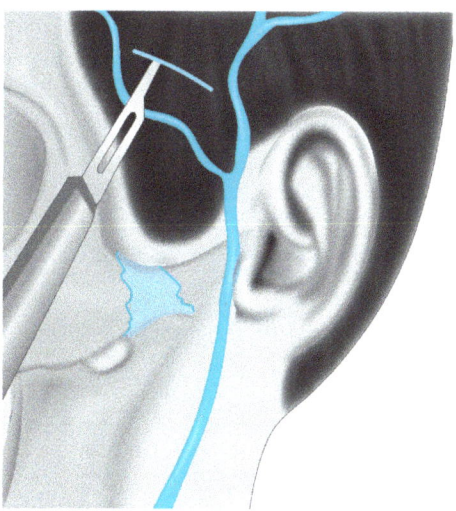

Fig. 7: Gillie's approach

Coronal incision: The coronal incision is ideal for exposure of the zygomatic arch, lateral orbital rim (frontozygomatic suture), lateral wall of the orbit (sphenozygomatic suture), and can also be used to harvest split calvarial bone graft.

Intraoral Incisions

Maxillary buccal sulcus approach (Balasubramaniam): The intraoral maxillary vestibular approach facilitates the exposure of the lateral buttress of the midface. It can also be used to expose the inferior orbital rim. The lateral maxillary vestibular approach can also be used to help reposition the depressed zygoma.

Lateral coronoid approach (Quin's): Through the intraoral incision, an instrument (Seldin retractor, urethral sound, and Henahan retractor) is placed between the coronoid process and the zygomatic arch. Lateral pressure is applied to the arch until the medially displaced arch is reduced.

ORBIT FRACTURES

There are three basic approaches through the external skin of the lower eyelid to give access to the inferior, lower medial, and lateral aspects of the orbital cavity (Fig. 8).
- Subciliary (A, synonym: lower blepharoplasty)
- Subtarsal (B, synonym: lower or mideyelid)
- Infraorbital (C, synonym: inferior orbital rim)
- The subciliary approach can be extended laterally to gain access to the lateral orbital rim (D).

The course of the incisions is aligned to the slope of the natural skin creases which become more apparent with age.

The skin of eyelid is the thinnest in the human body. It has little or no dermis and almost no subdermal fat.

Hypertrophic scarring and keloid formation is very uncommon following lower lid skin incisions. In general, the scars become inconspicuous with time.

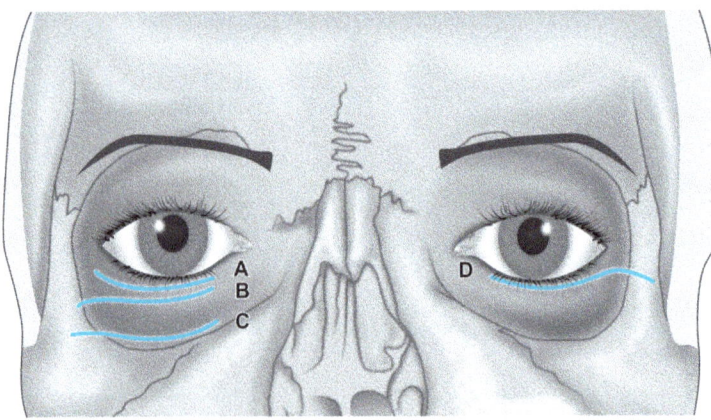

Fig. 8: Orbit fractures—Three basic approaches through the external skin: A—Subciliary, B—Subtarsal, C—Infraorbital, D—Subciliary approach extended laterally to gain access to the lateral orbital rim

There are other important incisions (Fig. 9). They are:
1. Stallard-Wright lateral orbitotomy incision
2. Lid crease with lateral extension
3. Modified Berke lateral canthotomy incision

4. Transcaruncular incision
5. Frontoethmoidal "Lynch" incision
6. Vertical lid split incision
7. Transconjunctival medial orbitotomy
8. Lateral canthotomy incision
9. Lower lid percutaneous incision
10. Transconjunctival lower lid incision.

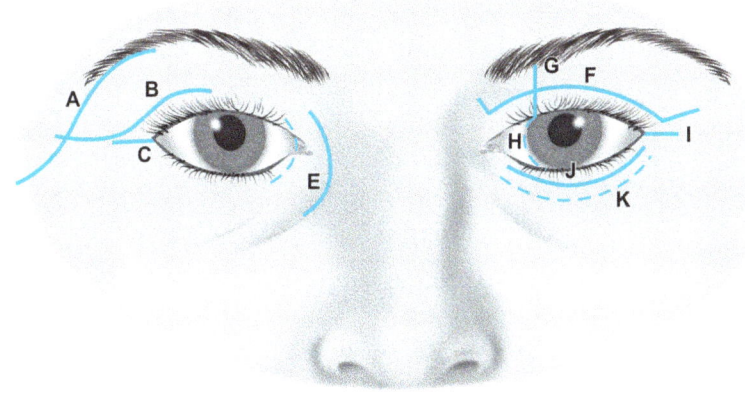

Fig. 9: Orbital incisions: (Posterior approach) A—Stallard-Wright lateral orbitotomy incision; B—lid crease with lateral extension; C—modified Berke lateral canthotomy incision; D— transcaruncular incision; E—frontoethmoidal "Lynch" incision. (Anterior approach) F—upper lid crease incision; G—vertical lid split incision; H, transconjunctival medial orbitotomy; I— lateral canthotomy incision; J—lower lid percutaneous incision; K—transconjunctival lower lid incision

FRONTAL BONE FRACTURES

The most common incision used for frontal bone fractures are as follows:
1. **Coronal Incision:** Hemicoronal (unilateral incision) and bicoronal or coronal incision (bilateral incision) is more extensive, but versatile surgical approach to the upper and middle regions of the facial skeleton, including the zygomatic arch and the TM joint areas. It provides excellent access to these areas with minimum complications.

    A major advantage is that most of the scars are hidden within the hairline, when the incision is extended into the preauricular area, the surgical scar is inconspicuous. This incision can be utilized for more extensive bilateral involvement.

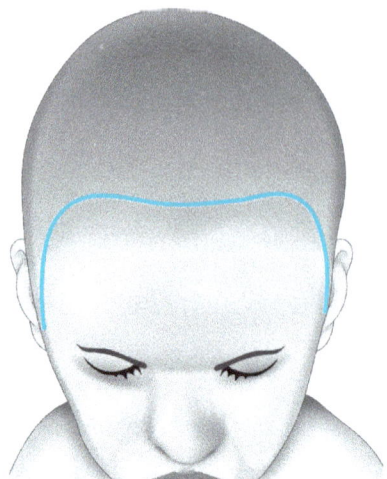

Fig. 10: Bicoronal incision

2. **Supraciliary Incision:** It is placed on the upper lid crease for base of frontal bone fractures near skull base (Fig. 9F).
3. **Existing lacerations:** Most of the times frontal bones fractures are accompanied by lacerations on forehead. Fractures of frontal bone can be approached by these lacerations.

NASO-ORBITO-ETHMOID FRACTURES

The following are the incisions for approaching Naso-orbito-ethmoidal fractures.
1. **Bicoronal incision:** Explained in above section (Fig. 10).
2. **Vertical incision (Stranc):** Midline incison on the nasal bone starting above the nasofrontal junction till the end of the nasal bone (Fig. 11).

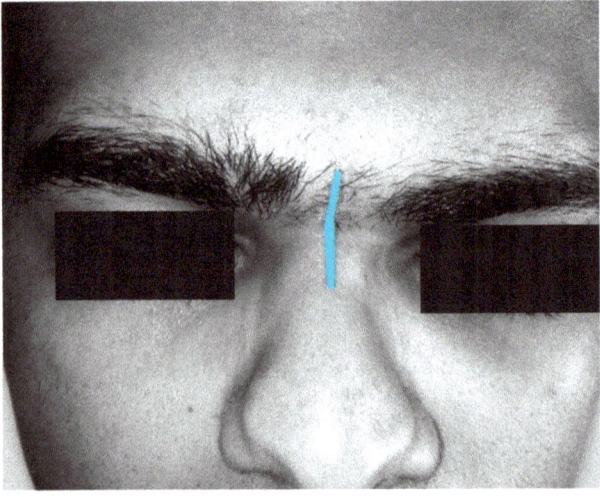

Fig. 11: Vertical incision (Stranc)

3. **Open sky approach (Converse and smith):** It is an H-shaped incision with two vertical limbs on either side of the nasal bone and a connecting incision placed in between them (Fig. 12).

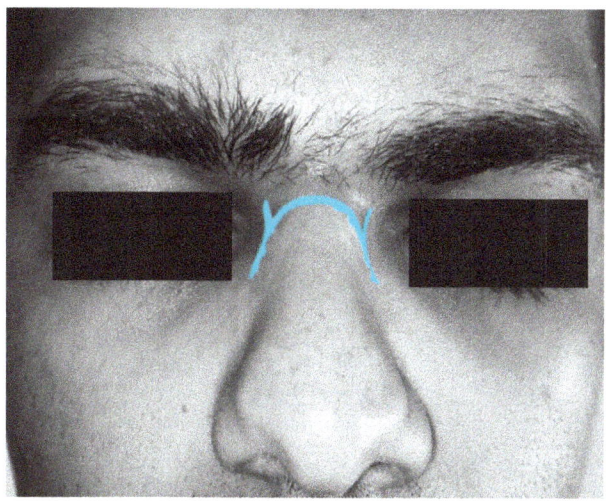

Fig. 12: Open sky approach (Converse and smith)

4. **Bowerman's incison:** It a W-shaped incision like a butterfly (Fig. 13).

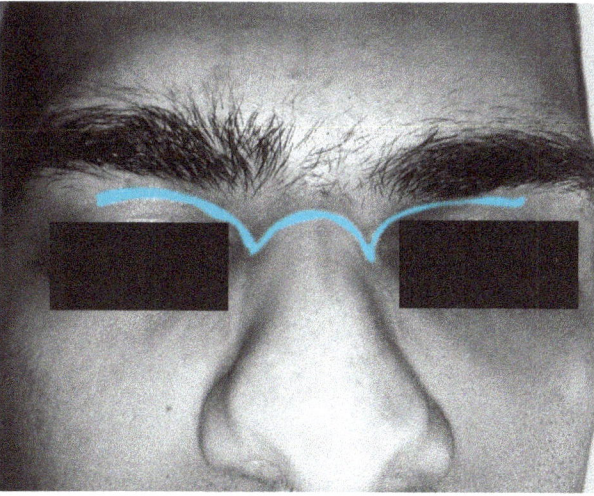

Fig. 13: Bowerman's incison

5. **Dingman incision:** It is bilateral Z-shaped incision on either side of nasal bone near the medical canthus (Fig. 14).
6. **Seagul incision:** It is a V-shaped incision placed above the supraciliary arches (Fig. 15).

7. **Transcaruncular incision:** Explained in above section "Orbit".
8. **Horizontal radix:** It is a straight horizontal line placed on just below the nasofrontal junction (Fig. 16).

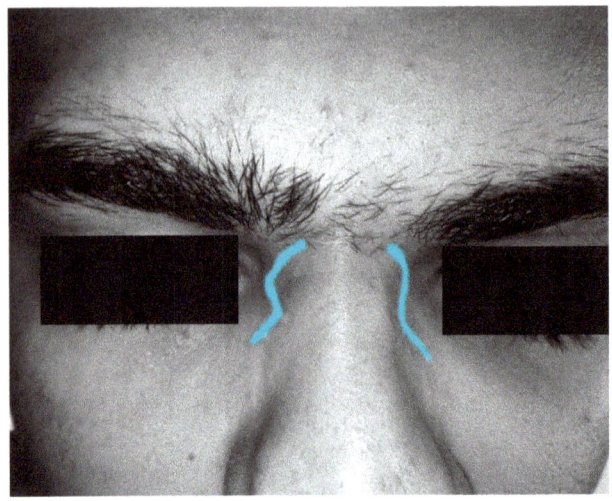

Fig. 14: Dingman incision

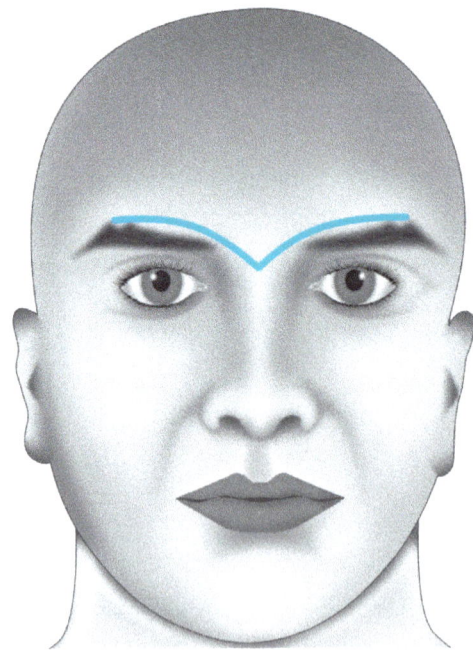

Fig. 15: Seagul incision

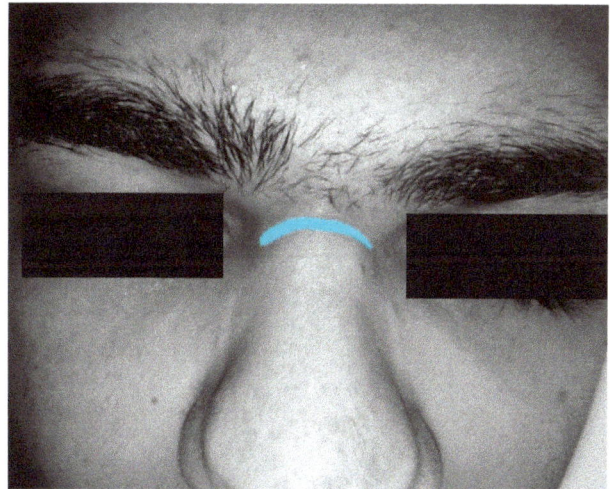

Fig. 16: Horizontal radix incision

9. **Existing laceration:** The fracture can be exposed by existing laceration.

CHAPTER

7

Space Infections

Incision Placement for Extraoral Drainage of Head and Neck Infections

Fascial spaces are the potential spaces between the fascia and the underlying vital organs/structures. Any infection between these fascia can cause spread of infections along the fascial planes.

Most common etiology in maxillofacial space infection is the dental infections leading to neck space infections. It may be as severe causing airway obstruction and hence emergency incision and drainage is required. The following incisions given in the Figure 1 below are used to drain space infections of different maxillofacial areas. All these are stab incisions placed with BP blade no 11 and corrugated rubber drain is kept for 2 days.

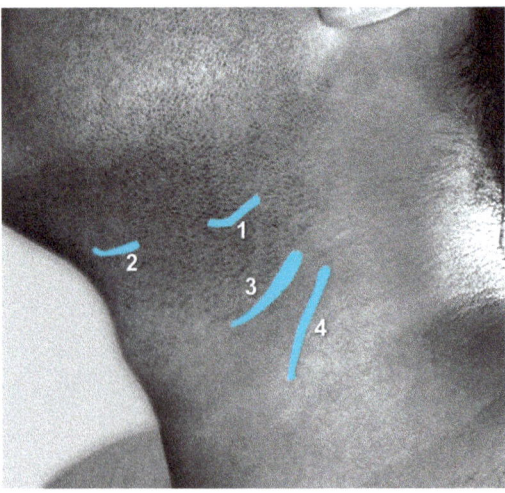

Fig. 1: Incision used to drain space infections of different maxillofacial areas

1. Incision given in neck crease to drain submandibular spaces, submental space, pterygomandibular and submasseteric space.
2. Incision given in submental area to drain submental and sublingual spaces.
3. Incision given in carotid triangle along the second neck crease to drain lateral pharyngeal and retropharyngeal spaces.
4. Incision given along the anterior border of sternomastoid muscle to drain lateral pharyngeal, retropharyngeal and carotid sheath space infections.

CHAPTER

8

Neoplasms

MAXILLARY NEOPLASMS

Removal of paranasal sinus tumors is a challenging exercise as far as the surgical planning and further reconstruction is concerned which may then be considered in three phases. First, one must assess the bony and soft tissue structures to be included for en bloc resection. Second, the approach must be designed to provide adequate exposure while preserving functional tissue and cosmetic integrity whenever possible. Third, the repair should be planned to use prosthetics or soft tissue techniques to best advantage. As far as radical maxillectomy is concerned, the classical Weber-Ferguson incision has been routinely used since age old times and still is being widely used due to its advantage of excellent exposure and minimal scarring as the incision follows the natural skin crease.

The following incisions are used for Maxillectomy:
- Low level maxillectomy: It can be approached by **Midfacial degloving approach (Fig. 1).**

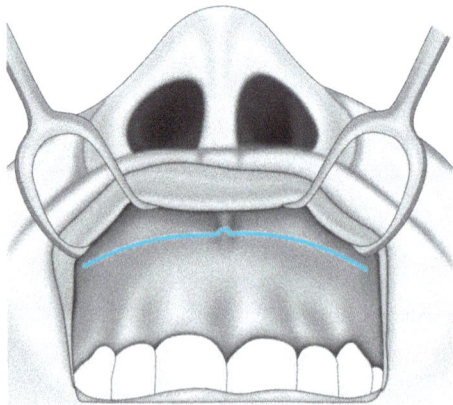

Fig. 1: Midfacial degloving approach

- High level or radical maxillectomy
    - **Lateral Rhinotomy:** On the nasal side, the tumor can be exposed via a lateral rhinotomy incision or endonasally with endoscopes
    - **Weber-Ferguson Incision:** The Weber-Ferguson approach is indicated to access for tumors involving the maxilla extending superiorly to the infraorbital nerve and into or involving the orbit. It provides a wide access to all areas of the maxilla and orbital floor (Fig. 2).

Modifications

- Lynch—Extending along the medial canthus
- Subciliary (Crocketts)—Extending below the eyelid
- Supraciliary—Extending above the eyelid
- Altemir—Incison along the philtral crest but not in the midline
- Lateral canthotomy—Extending along the lateral canthus
- Nasal rotation—Extending across the contralateral nose
- Borle's extention for maxillectomy. This incision helps to reconstruct the maxillectomy defect by temporalis muscle flap (Fig. 3).

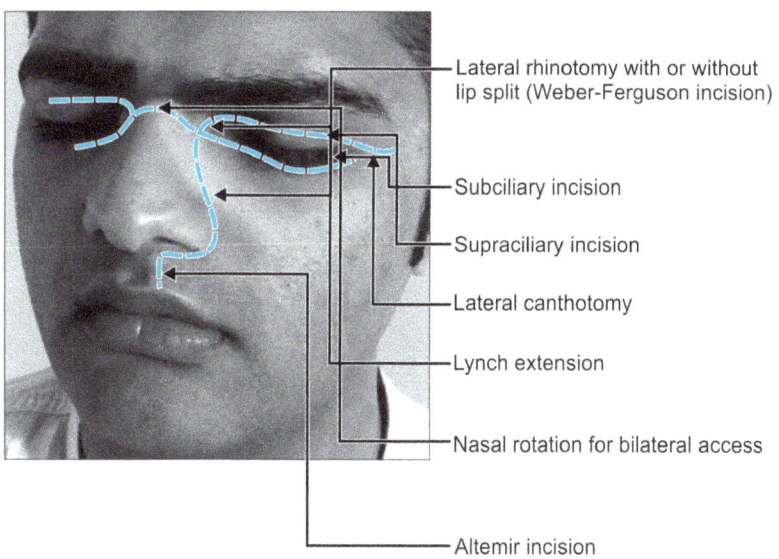

Fig. 2: Weber-Fergusson incision and its modifications

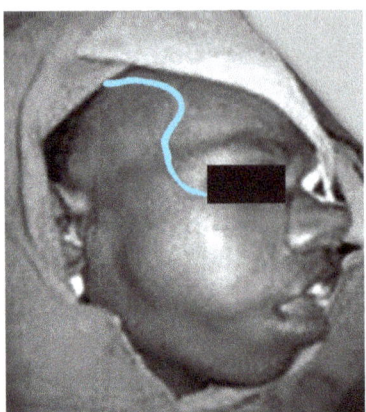

Fig. 3: Borle's extension for maxillectomy

Source: Borle et al. Modified Weber-Ferguson incision with Borle's extension, BJOMS, 48(5): e23-4, 2010

Modified Incision

(Kranti et al. Indian J Otolaryngol Head Neck Surg (April–June 2012) 64(2):184–187; DOI 10.1007/s12070-011-0143-8)

It consists of two separate incisions to provide better cosmetic result.

Eye Incision

First local infiltration is given at both medial and lateral canthus of eye. Then a lateral "Z-shaped" incision of about 1 cm is given at the lateral canthus and the medial canthus. These two incisions are joined together by incising conjunctiva in the lower fornix. For this purpose stay sutures are passed at each end of tarsal plate. Lower lid is then pulled outwards and downwards thereby exposing the conjunctival fornix which can then be incised. Incision is then deepened to the bone incising periosteum at inferior orbital margin. Periosteum is elevated over the inferior orbital plate as well as on the anterolateral wall of maxilla and root of zygoma.

Midface Degloving Incision

A midface degloving incisions are given and on the side of the lesion the incision is extended behind the maxillary tuberosity.

MANDIBULAR/ORAL CAVITY NEOPLASMS

Lip Splitting Incisions

The use of a lip splitting incision with a lateral extension into the neck incision allows for the elevation of a cheek flap and exposure of the hemimandible and oral cavity.

Neoplasms | 29

- **Roux-Trotter incision:** Incision in midline of lip and chin (Fig. 4)

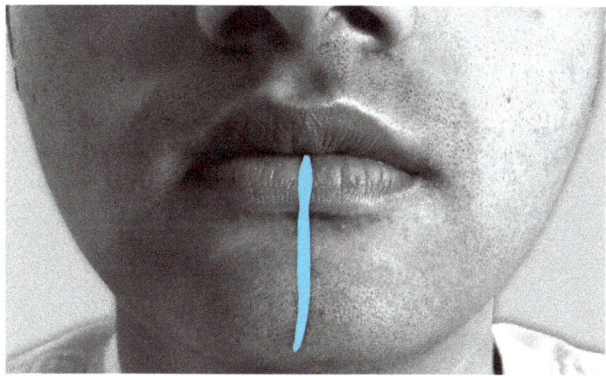

Fig. 4: Roux-Trotter incision

- **Robson incision or von Langenbeck incision:** Incision from the corner of lip along the labiomental fold (Fig. 5)

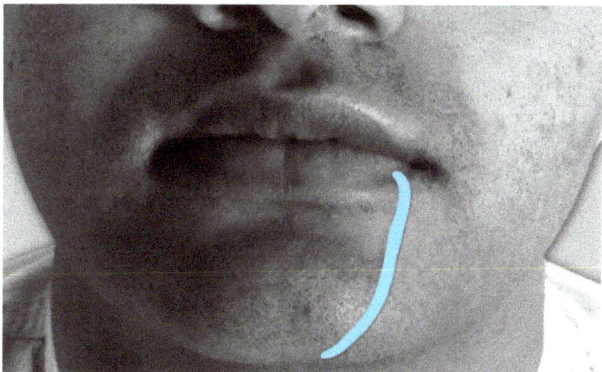

Fig. 5: Robson incision or von Langenbeck incision

- **McGregor incision:** Incision from midline of lip along the chin pad's convex contour (Fig. 6)

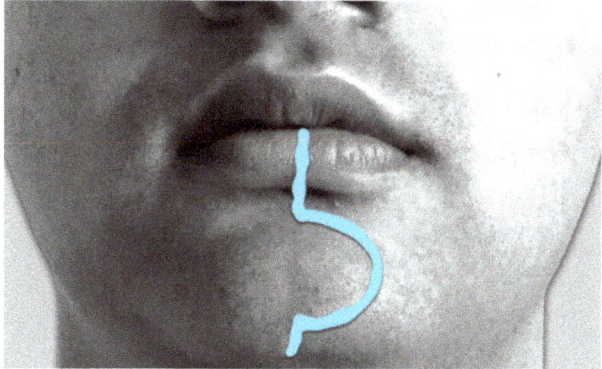

Fig. 6: McGregor incision

- **Hayter incision:** Same as McGregor incision with inclusion of a chevron in midline of lip incision (Fig. 7).

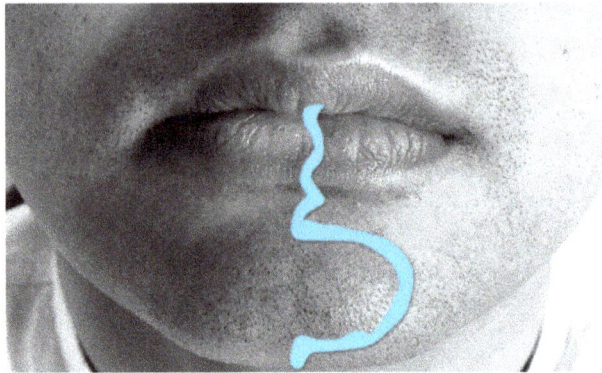

Fig. 7: Hayter incision

Modifications

- **Commisure split:** Incision from the angle of the lip along the convex contour of the chin reaching slightly lateral to midline of the chin and then joining the submandibular incision (Fig. 8)

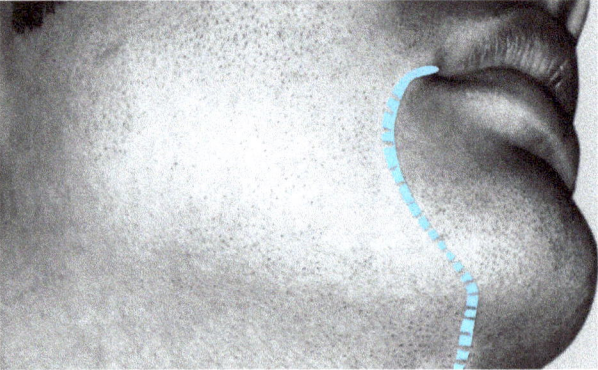

Fig. 8: Commisure split

- **Modified lip split incision (Fig. 9).**

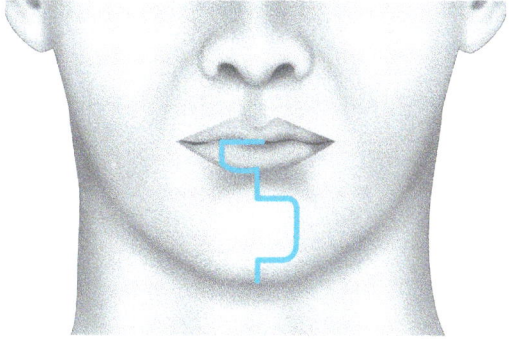

Fig. 9: Modified lip-split incision

Source: Bhatt, Vyomesh et al. Journal of Oral and Maxillofacial Surgery, Volume 67, Issue 1, 229–230

Neck Incisions

- **Submandibular incision:** This is the most commonly used incision in combination with any of the above lip splitting incisions to gain access to mandibular tumors or other oral cavity tumors like buccal mucosa/tongue/floor of mouth and retromolar trigone. This is placed in any crease of the neck usually first crease or 2 cm below the lower border of mandible to avoid inadvertent damage to marginal mandibular nerve (4th branch of facial nerve)
- **Visor incision:** This approach allows access to virtually any area of the oral cavity or oropharynx but, does require the release and pull through of advanced oromandibular tumors into the neck (Fig. 10)

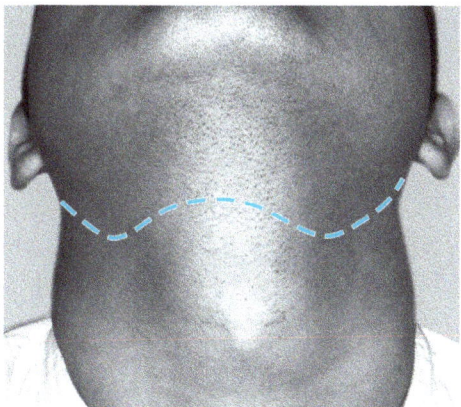

Fig. 10: Visor incision

- **Cheek Incisions:**
    - Burbosa incision
    - Crokett's incision
    - Jaegar Jugal incision.

Infratemporal Fossa Approach Incision

- **Preauricular with lazy 'S' incision:** The presence of neurovascular structures within the infratemporal fossa (ITF) (e.g. ICA) or adjacent to it (e.g. CN VII) is the limiting step for designing a surgical approach to the ITF. Surgical approaches often center on the preservation and identification of these neurovascular entities (Figs 11A and B)
- **Fish Type 'A' approach (Transtemporal) (Fig. 12).**

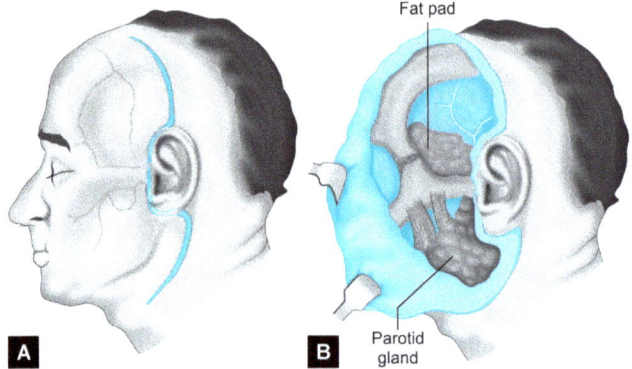

Figs 11A and B: Preauricular with lazy 'S' incision: (A) Bicoronal scalp incision is extended along preauricular skin crease. This incision may be continued into upper cervical region as a lazy S incision, or a separate cervical incision may be made for exposure of vessels and nerves; (B) Scalp flap is elevated from underlying cranium, fascia, lateral orbital rim, zygomatic arch, and masseteric fascia. Plane of dissection is deep to superficial layer of deep temporal fascia (incised) and deep to parotid masseteric fascia

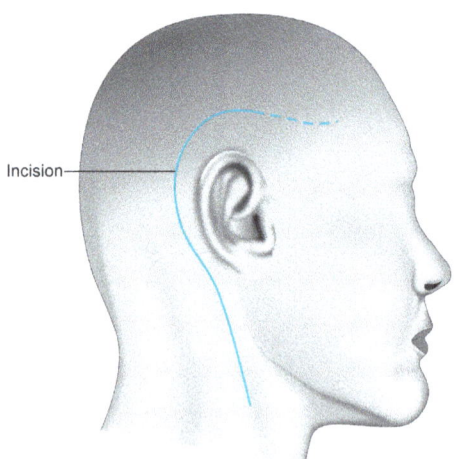

Fig. 12: Fish type 'A' approach

NECK DISSECTIONS

Lymphadenectomy (Fig. 13) is the surgical removal of one or more groups of lymph nodes. It is almost always performed as part of the surgical management of cancer. Neck dissection is done to remove the group of cervical lymph nodes (Level I – VI). There are numerous incisions for neck dissection. Some of them are given below.

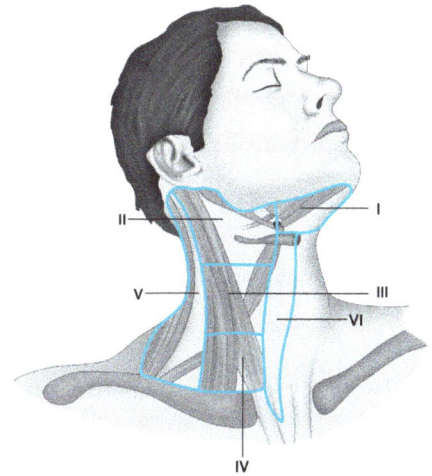

Fig. 13: Lymphadenectomy

Supraomohyoid Neck Dissection

Supraomohyoid neck dissection (SOHND) involves removal of cervical lymph nodes from level I–III (Figs 14A to D).

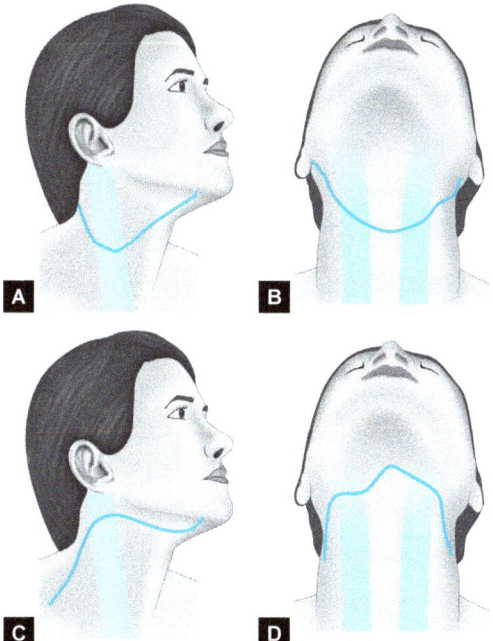

Figs 14A to D: Supraomohyoid neck dissection: (A) Modified apron incision; (B) Apron incision; (C) Boomerang incision; (D) Bilateral boomerang incision

Modified Radical Neck Dissection

Modified radical neck dissection (MRND) involves removal of lymph node levels I–V with preservation of at least one of the nonlymphatic structures (spinal accessory nerve, internal jugular vein, or sternocleidomastoid).

Radical Neck Dissection

Radical neck dissection (RND) involve removal of lymph node levels I–V, the spinal accessory nerve, internal jugular vein, and sternocleidomastoid.

Hockey Stick Incision (Fig. 15)

Starts along the posterior border of sternocleidomastoid (STM) muscle reaching the clavicular head 2 cm above the clavicle and horizontal re-easing incision to raise the flap anteriorly.

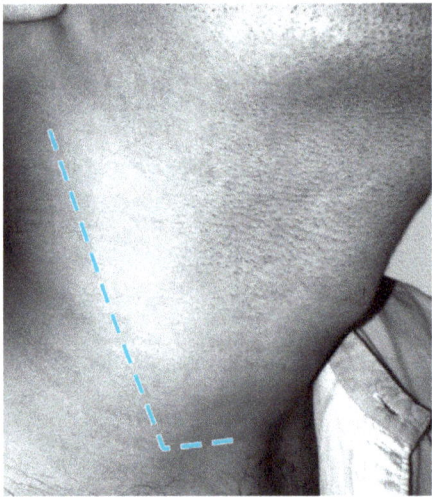

Fig. 15: Hockey stick incision

Boomerang Incision (Fig. 16)

Horizontal incision starts from the submental area, 1 cm from the mentum along the neck crease going posteriorly up to the posterior border of STM and then vertical incision in the form of "S" shape running down in the posterior triangle.

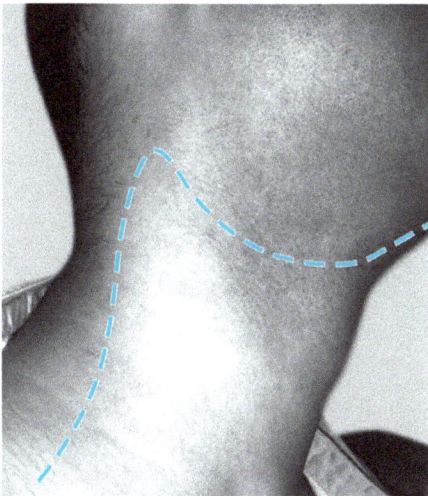

Fig. 16: Boomerang incision

McFee Incision (Fig. 17)

Two parallel incisions. First incision along the neck crease 2 cm below the lower border of mandible and the second incision of 3–4 cm, 2 cm above the clavicle in neck crease to expose the clavicular head of STM.

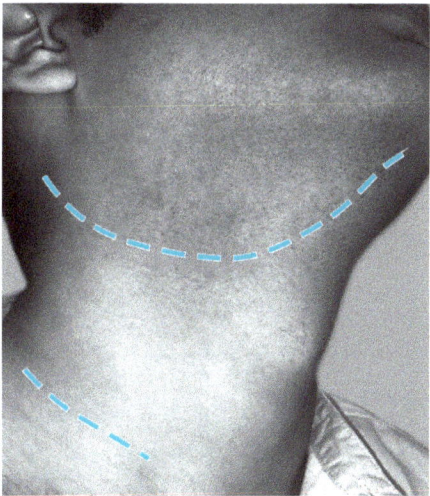

Fig. 17: McFee incision

George Crile Incision (Fig. 18)

Submandibular incision along the neck crease 2 cm below the lower border of mandible. Then vertical "S-shaped" incision is made from the center of submandibular incision.

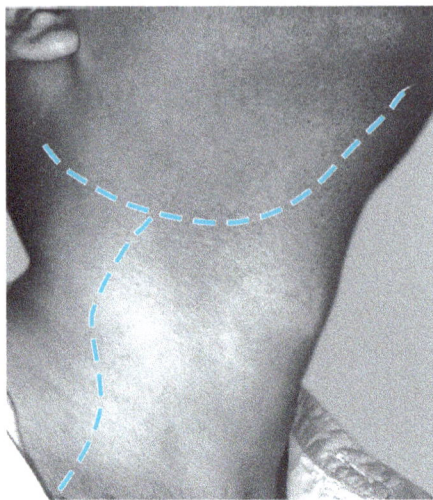

Fig. 18: George crile incision

Modified Schobinger Incision (Fig. 19)

Submandibular incision along the neck crease 2 cm below the lower border of mandible. Vertical "S-shaped" incision is dropped from the distal 3rd of sumandibular incision.

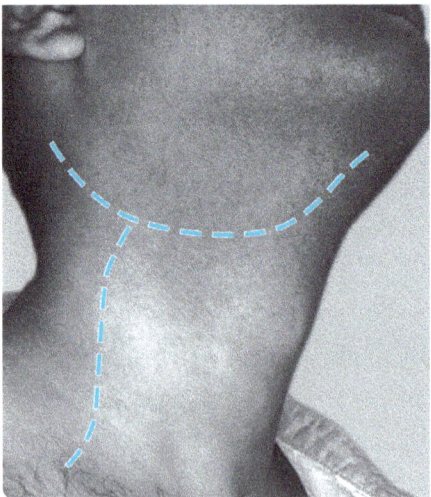

Fig. 19: Modified Schobinger incision

Bilateral Hockey Incision (Fig. 20)

The hockey stick incision is the standard incision that allows exposure of levels I through IV, but the Boomerang and McFee incisions also allow appropriate exposure while avoiding trifurcations (especially over the carotid). The

Boomerang incision is less aesthetically pleasing, but it can be extended through the mentum and lip for oral cavity tumors requiring a mandibulotomy.

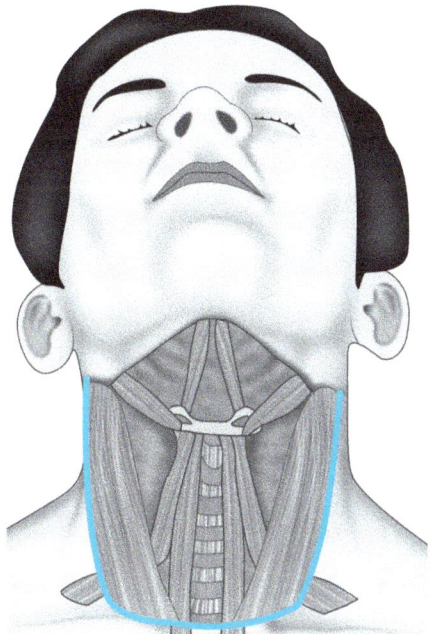

Fig. 20: Bilateral hockey incision

Conley Incision (Fig. 21)

Submandibular incision along the neck crease 2 cm below the lower border of mandible. Vertical straight incision running downwards and backwards from the center of submandibular incision.

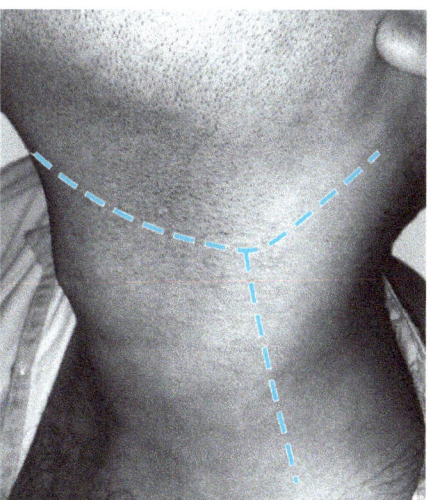

Fig. 21: Conley incision

Hetter's Incision (Fig. 22)

H-shaped incision. Two vertical curved incision with a center horizontal incision joining both incisions.

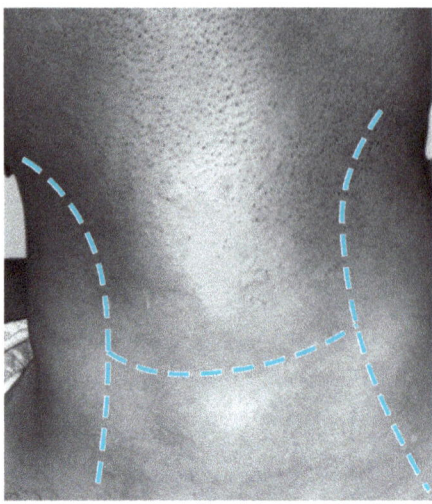

Fig. 22: Hetter's Incision

Other Incisions

There are numerous other incisions of neck dissection which are of historical significance rather than surgical significance. They are as follows (Fig. 23):

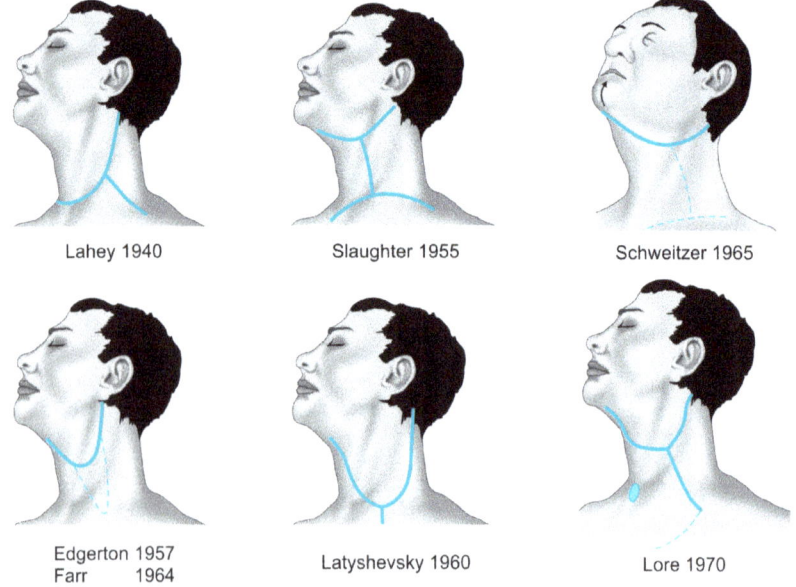

Fig. 23: Other incisions

INCISIONS FOR SALIVARY GLAND NEOPLASM

Incisions for salivary gland neoplasms are discussed below. Parotidectomy is the removal of part or all of the parotid gland on one side of the face.

- **Traditional parotidectomy incision or lazy 'S' incision:** The traditional parotidectomy was performed through a modified Blair incision in which an incision was made from the top of the ear down toward the jaw and was several inches in length. The entire side of the face is then pulled back to allow for visualization of the entire area, including the facial nerve (Fig. 24)

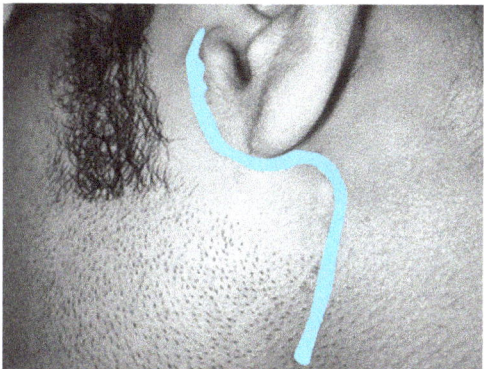

Fig. 24: Traditional parotidectomy incision or lazy 'S' incision

- **Mini-parotid incision:** The small incision reduces scarring under the surface and therefore has long-term complications, as well as provide patients with a shorter recovery time (Fig. 25)

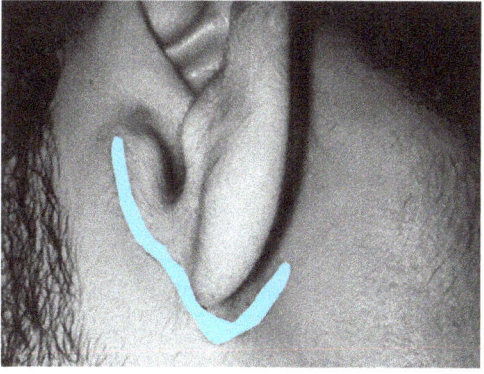

Fig. 25: Mini-parotid incision

- **Facelift incision:** The use of a facelift incision results in less scarring than the traditional modified Blair incision and a better aesthetic outcome. This incision allows for good access to the facial nerve, greater auricular nerve and the SCM muscle to be used for reconstruction (Fig. 26)

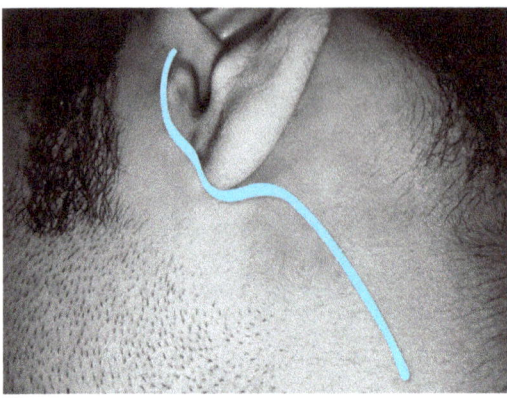

Fig. 26: Facelift incision

- **Modified Blair's incision:** The preauricular incision is made in the preauricular crease and extended down along the neck crease. Similar to lazy 'S' incision
- **Retroauricular incision:** Incision behind the ear (Fig. 27)

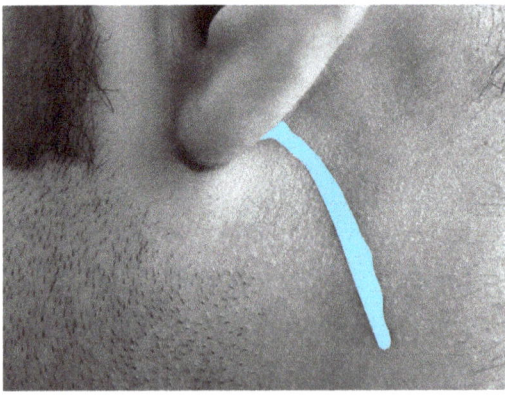

Fig. 27: Retroauricular incision

- **Submandibular incision:** This incision can be placed on first crease of neck to remove submandibular gland
- **Intraoral incision:** A linear incision may be placed in floor of mouth lateral to tongue to remove deep portion of submandibular gland and sublingual gland.

THYROID TUMORS

A thyroidectomy is the surgical removal of all or part of the thyroid gland. It is usually performed when a patient has thyroid cancer or some other condition of the thyroid gland, such as hyperthyroidism or goiter. There can be other indications like cosmesis or any kind of symptomatic obstruction causing airway difficulty.

Thyroidectomy incisions have traditionally been placed using a long-curved incision called as a necklace incision at the base of the neck, either just above or below the clavicle. This approach is still used by most surgeons as it is traditionally what was taught, but there are now alternative approaches. The base of neck approach still requires a longer incision than alternatives as more dissection is required to reach the thyroid which is actually quite high in the neck. Alternatives include the extra cervical approaches where the incision is not in the neck at all, the mini-incision cervical approaches for small thyroid nodules, and the high cricoid approach for larger nodules and goiters (Fig. 28).

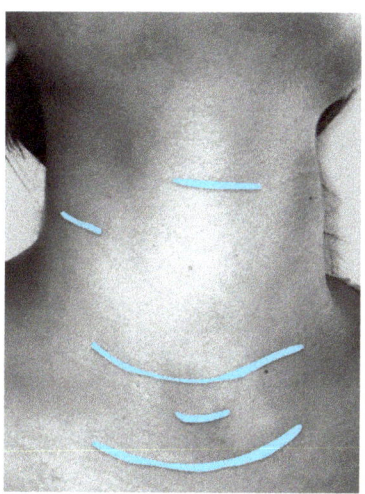

Fig. 28: Three smaller incisions—Mini incisions, Larger incision—Necklace incision

Transaxillary Thyroidectomy by Da Vinci Robotic System

Transaxillary thyroidectomy is a minimally invasive surgical technique to remove all or part of the thyroid (Fig. 29).

The incision is 5–7 cm long, but it is hidden—not in front and center, like neck scars from open or even most endoscopic thyroidectomies. There is another very small incision—5 mm in the chest.

Robotic thyroidectomy is done using the da Vinci Surgical System, a system that's been used in many other robot-assisted surgeries with much success. The da Vinci system has:
- Four robotic hands: These are called EndoWrist instruments, and they do work just like hands. They can grab things, twist, and turn—and they're incredibly small. The robotic hands allow the surgeon to make very precise movements

- 3D camera: This is a high-definition camera that gives the surgeon a 3D image of the thyroid. He or she can zoom in and get an even more detailed look; the camera includes magnification of 10x
- Console: The surgeon sits at the console, where he or she controls the four robotic hands and sees images from the 3D camera.

The four robotic hands and the 3D camera are inserted through the incisions. The surgeon can then accurately remove part or all of the thyroid, depending on what the patient needs.

Axillary Incision

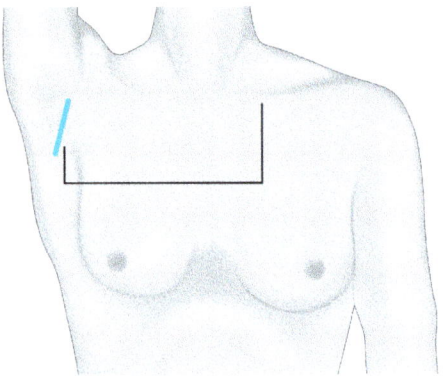

Fig. 29: Transaxillary thyroidectomy

Laryngeal Tumors

Total laryngectomy is a surgical procedure to remove the larynx when the patient has a neoplasm. The incision used for laryngectomy is called as Gluck-Sorenson which is a U-shaped incision (Fig. 30).

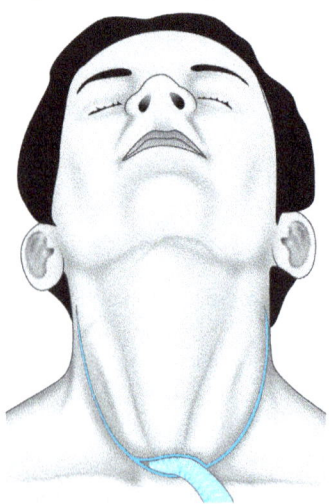

Fig. 30: Gluck–Sorenson incision

Lymph Node Excisions/Lateral Neck Swellings

Incision for lateral neck swelling like lymph nodes or any other neck swellings is placed in the neck crease in inconspicuous areas.

Incision for carotid body tumor is placed obliquely more or less parallel to the anterior border of sternomastoid muscle or can also be placed as horizontal incision in the neck crease (Fig. 31).

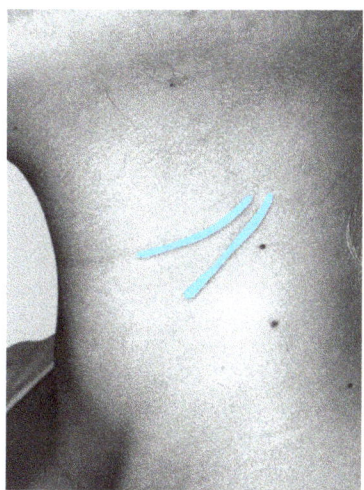

Fig. 31: Carotid body tumor incision line

CHAPTER

9

Cleft Lip

Cleft lip is a congenital split in the upper lip on one or both sides at the philtral region, often associated with a cleft palate.

CLEFT LIP INCISIONS

Millard Rotation—Advancement flap (Unilateral)

The steps are described in Figures 1A to E.

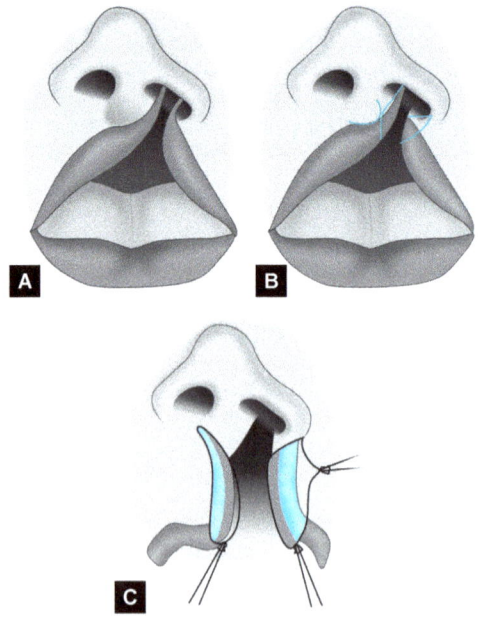

Figs 1A to E: *Contd..*

Cleft Lip

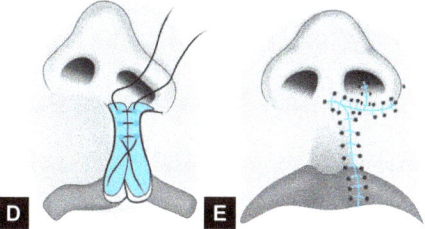

Figs 1A to E: Millard rotation—advancement flap (Unilateral) (A) Complete unilateral cleft of the lip. (B) Markings of the incisions based on the need to excise the hypoplastic tissue and approximate good vermilion and white roll tissue for the repair. (C) Once the hypoplastic tissue has been excised, the three layers of tissue are dissected (skin, muscle, and mucosa). The orbicularis muscle must be completely free from its abnormal insertions on the anterior nasal spine area and lateral alar base. (D) The orbicularis oris muscle is approximated with multiple interrupted sutures, and the vermilion border/white roll complex is reconstructed with approximation of the nasal floor and mucosal flaps. (E) The lateral flap is advanced and the medial segment is rotated downward to create a healing scarline that will resemble the natural philtral column on the opposite side

Millard Rotation—Advancement Flap (Bilateral)

The steps are described in Figures 2A to E.

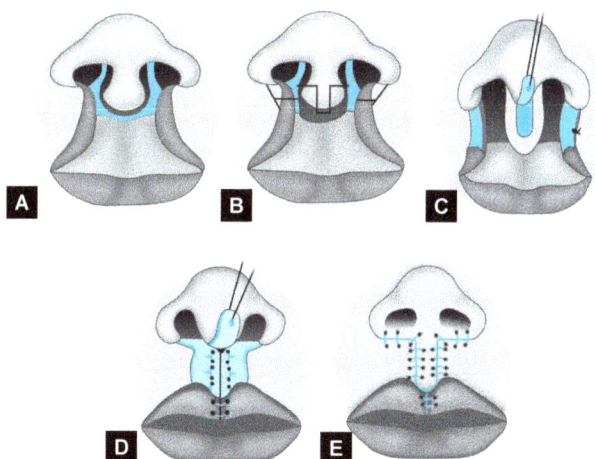

Figs 2A to E: Millard rotation—advancement flap (bilateral) (A) Complete bilateral cleft of the lip and maxilla. (B) Markings of the incisions with emphasis on excision of hypoplastic tissue and approximating more normal tissue with the advancement flaps. (C) A new philtrum is created by excising the lateral hypoplastic tissue and elevating the philtrum superiorly. (D) The orbicularis oris musculature is approximated in the midline with multiple interrupted and/or mattress sutures. There is no musculature present in the premaxillary segment, and this must be brought to the midline from each lateral advancement flap with the nasal floor flaps sutured at this time. The new vermillion border is reconstructed in the midline with good white-roll tissue advanced from the lateral flaps. (E) Final approximation of the skin and mucosal tissues is performed

Tenison-Randall Flap (Triangular Flap)

Tenison-Randal flap is shown in Figures 3A and B.

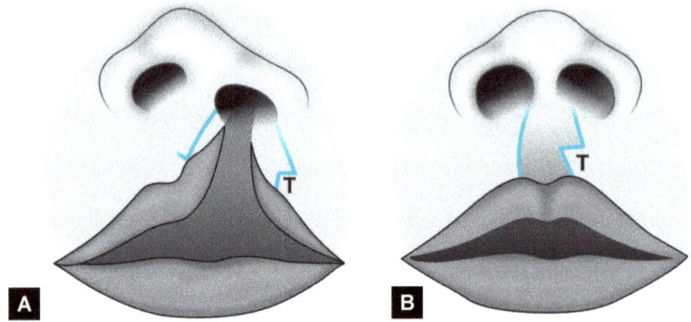

Figs 3A and B: Tenison-Randall flap

Other Incisions (Fig. 4)

- V Excision
- von Graefe
- Malgaigne
- Rose
- Thompson
- Koenig
- Hagedorn
- Le Mesurier
- Collis
- Mirault
- Brown McDowell
- Tennison
- Skoog
- Millard.

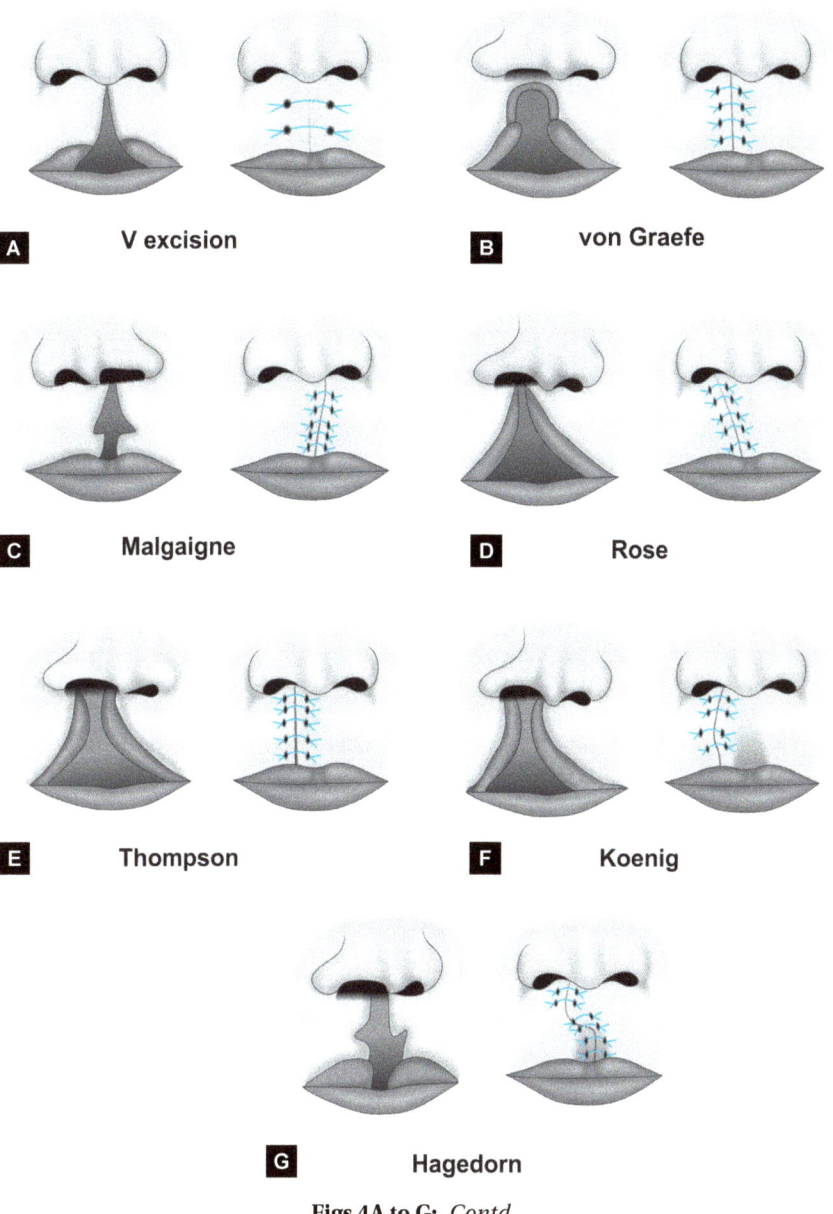

Figs 4A to G: *Contd...*

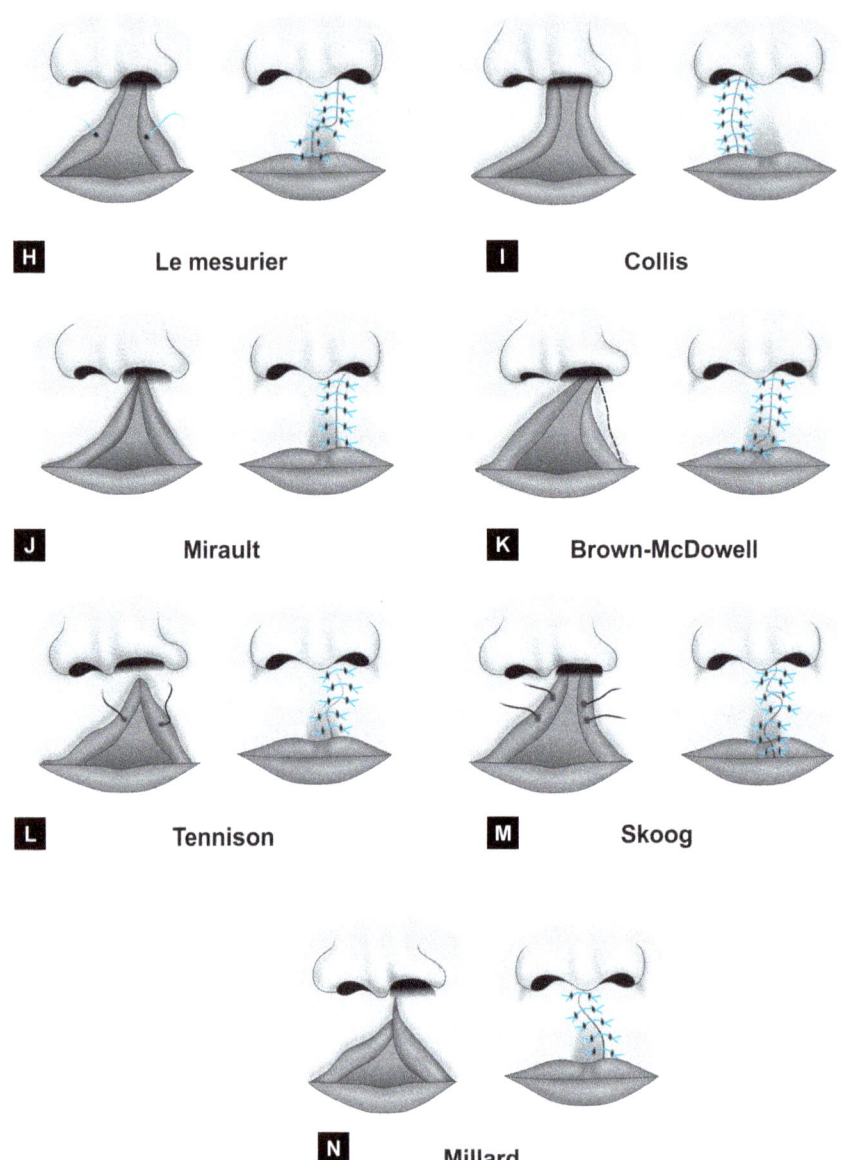

Figs 4H to N: Other incisions

CHAPTER
10

Cleft Palate

Bardach Palatoplasty

The process of Bardach Palatoplasty is described in Figures 1A to D.

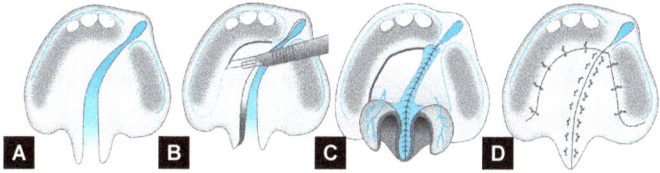

Figs 1A to D: Bardach Palatoplasty: (A) Unilateral cleft of the primary and secondary palates extending to the uvula. (B) Two large full-thickness mucoperiosteal flaps are elevated from each palate shelf. (C) A layered closure is performed. The muscle bellies of the levator palatini are elevated off of their abnormal insertions on the posterior palate. They are then approximated in the midline to create a dynamic functional sling for speech purposes. (D) Once the nasal mucosa and musculature of the soft palate are approximated, the oral mucosa is closed in the midline. The lateral releasing incisions are quite easily closed primarily due to the length gained from the depth of the palate

Furlow Z-plasty

The steps of Furlow Z-plasty are described in Figures 2A to D.

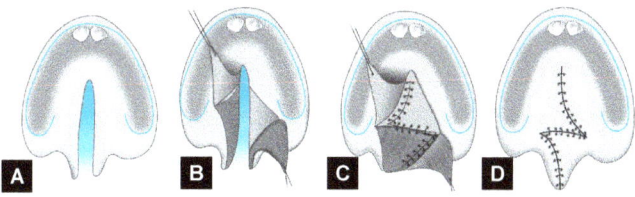

Figs 2A to D: Furlow Z-plasty: (A) Cleft of the secondary palate (both hard and soft) from the incisive foramen to the uvula. (B) Z-plasty flaps developed on the oral and then nasal side. (C) The flaps are then transposed to lengthen the soft palate. A nasal side closure is completed in the standard fashion anterior to the junction of the hard and soft palate. (D) The oral side flaps are then transposed and closed in a similar fashion completing the palate closure

Von Langenbeck Palatoplasty

The steps in the process of von Langenbeck Palatoplasty are described in Figures 3A to C.

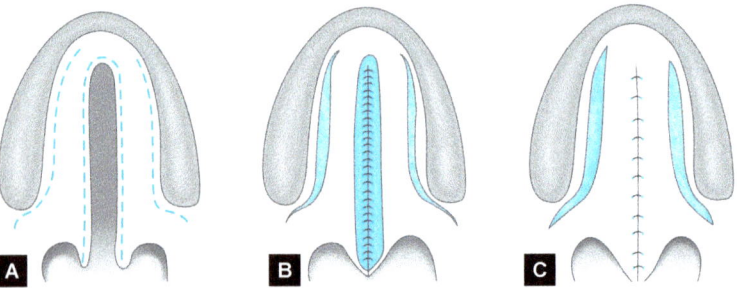

Figs 3A to C: von Langenbeck Palatoplasty: (A) Unilateral cleft of the primary and secondary palates extending to the uvula. (B) Two large full-thickness mucoperiosteal flaps are elevated from each palate shelf. (C) A layered closure is performed. The muscle bellies of the levator palatini are elevated off of their abnormal insertions on the posterior palate. They are then approximated in the midline to create a dynamic functional sling for speech purposes

CHAPTER
11

Temporomandibular Joint

The following incisions are used for approach of Temporomandibular joint (TMJ) for neoplasms and condylar fractures.
Ideally, the selected approach should accomplish the following:
- Maximize exposure for the specific procedure
- Avoid damage to the branches of the facial nerve
- Avoid damage to major vessels (e.g. internal maxillary artery, retromandibular vein)
- Avoid damage to the parotid gland
- Maximize use of natural skin creases for cosmetic wound closure.

INCISIONS

- Preauricular
    - Dingman's incision
    - Blair's incision
    - Thoma's incision
    - Al-Kayat and Bramley's incision
    - Popowich's modification of Al-Kayat and Bramley's.
- Endaural incision
- Postauricular incision
- Rhytidectomy incision
- Submandibular (Risdon's approach)
- Postramal (Hind's approach)
- Trans-tragal incision
- Coronal or bicoronal approach
- Intraoral incision.

Preauricular Approach (Fig. 1)

The preauricular approach is one of the most commonly used to expose the TMJ. The incision starts in front of the ear at the level of attachment of the auricle and follows the anterior border of the ear until it reaches the point of attachment of the lobule.

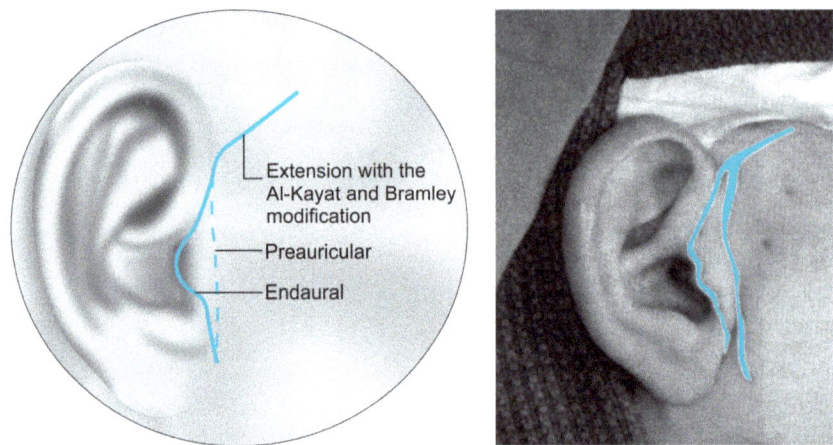

Fig. 1: Preauricular approach

A preauricular, endaural incision is divided into three parts (Fig. 2):
1. The curvilinear superior aspect from the top of the pinna to the top of the tragus.
2. The prelobular section in the most convenient crease from the inferior aspect of the tragus to the lowest level of the lobe.
3. The endaural portion, which connects the first two incisions from the skin crease just above the tragus to the skin crease just below it.

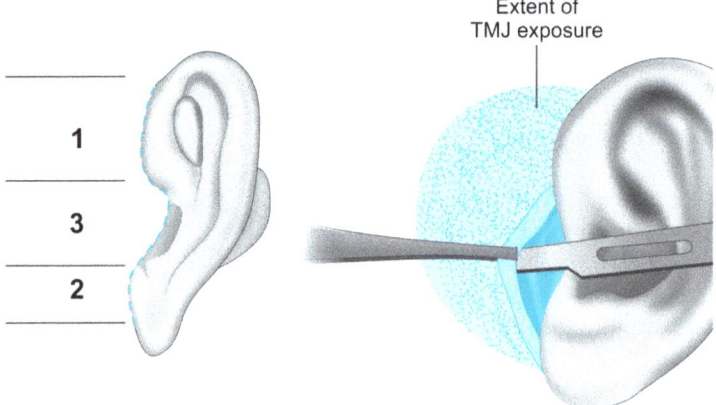

Fig. 2: Parts of preauricular incision

Modifications of Basic Preauricular Incision

All these modifications of basic preauricular incision were made to have better access and visibility, and wider exposure and to prevent injury to the auriculotemporal nerve and the branches of dying facial nerve (Figs 3 and 4).

- Blair and Ivy in 1936 used an 'inverted hockey stick' incision over the zygomatic arch, which gave easy access and better visibility and also facilitated exposure of the arch along with condylar area
- Thoma in 1958—recommended an 'angulated vertical incision' which is carried out across the zygomatic arch in the fold, directly in front of the ear, extending down slightly above the ear lobe, to avoid the main trunk of the facial nerve
- Al-Kayat and Bramley in 1979 described a modified preauricular approach to TMJ and zygomatic arch considering the main branches of the vessels and nerves in the viscinity
- Popowich and Crane in 1982 further modified basic Al-Kayat and Bramley's incision. A large incision shaped like question mark was made in the temporal area and extended in the preauricular area.

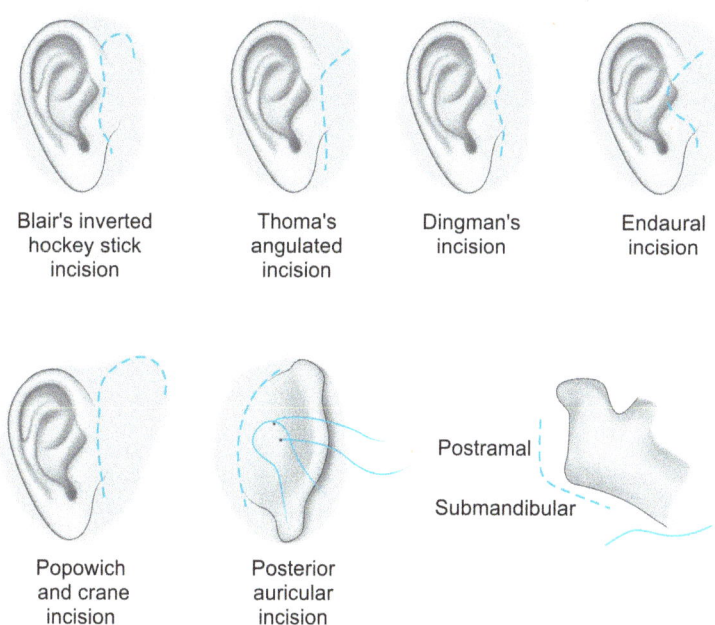

Fig. 3: Modifications of preauricular incision

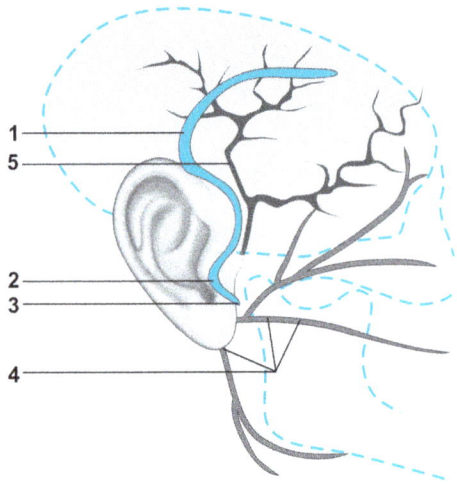

Fig. 4: Modified preauricular incision—(1) skin incision; (2) tragus, (3) lower limit of skin incision; (4) facial nerve branches; (5) superficial temporal artery

Endaural Approach (Fig. 5)

Rongetti described a modification of Lempert's endaural approach to the mastoid process for surgical improvement of otosclerosis, for approaching the TMJ. The endaural incisions employed today either incorporate the anterior wall of the external auditory canal, or the tragus, or simply the skin overlying the mental aspect of the tragus.

The incision begins well within the external auditory meatus at the superior mental wall. At this level, the incision is made down to the bone and extended in a curvilinear fashion upward hugging the anterior helix. It becomes less penetrating as it approaches the superior surface, ending at about the level of the inferior tragus. The incision is deepened to the level of the temporalis fascia. The incision is now continued inferiorly, with the knife in continuous contact with the tympanic plate, to make a semicircular incision to the inferior point of the meatus. The incision is then continued anteroinferiorly to fall into the incisura-intertragica, ending just before it approaches the surface. The application of forward traction on the inner aspect of the tragus assists the surgeon in completing the incision. Sharp dissection is carried deeply for some distance along the perichondrium. The flap is then reflected en masse anteroinferiorly off the lateral capsule and ligament.

Postauricular Approach (Fig. 6)

In the postauricular approach, the incision is made posterior to the ear and involves the sectioning of the external auditory meatus. Excellent posterolateral exposure is afforded with this technique. The flap, once reflected, contains the entire auricle and superficial lobe of the parotid gland.

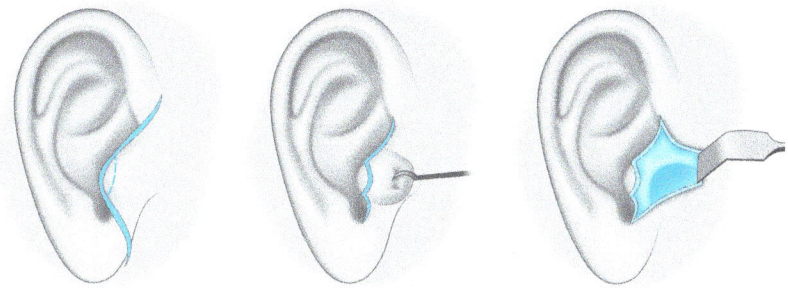

Fig. 5: Endaural approach

The incision in the postauricular approach begins near the superior aspect of the external pinna and is extended to the tip of the mastoid process. The superior portion may be extended obliquely into the hairline for additional exposure. The incision is made 3-5 mm parallel and posterior to the postauricular flexure.

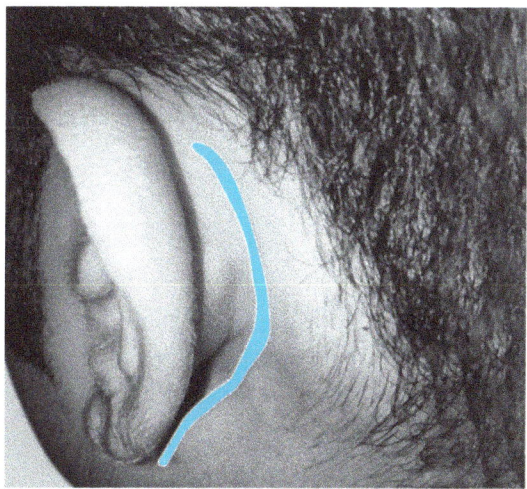

Fig. 6: Postauricular approach

The advantages of the postauricular approach lie in the predictability of the anatomic exposure. Dissection to the joint is rapid with minimal bleeding. The approach offers an alternative for a patient who has had previous procedures in this region. This approach may not be desirable in the patient susceptible to keloid formation, owing to the potential for a keloid to develop in the meatus. Meatal atresia has been reported with this technique. The risk of facial nerve injury is not eliminated.

Submandibular (Risdon's) Approach (Fig. 7)

Because of its distant location from the TMJ, this approach provides the poorest access to the region. However, it can be used for open reduction of low subcondylar fractures and as part of the approach for the placement of condylar prostheses and grafts, although the retromandibular incision provides better access and results in a more aesthetic, less obvious scar.

The initial incision, which is about 3.0 cm long, is made through the skin and subcutaneous tissues to the level of the platysma muscle. It is placed either 1.0 or 2.0 cm below and parallel to the lower border of the mandible or slightly lower so that it is located in or parallel to a skin crease. The lower location generally produces a less conspicuous scar.

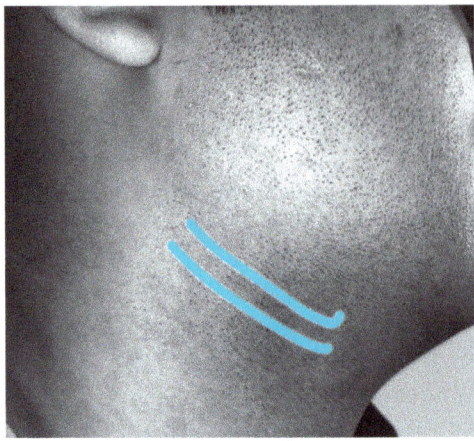

Fig. 7: Submandibular approach

Retromandibular/Postramal/Hind's Approach (Fig. 8)

A 3.0–3.5 cm incision is made through the skin and subcutaneous tissues just posterior and parallel to the posterior border of the ascending ramus, extending from a point just below the level of the lobule of the ear inferiorly to a point just above the angle of the mandible.

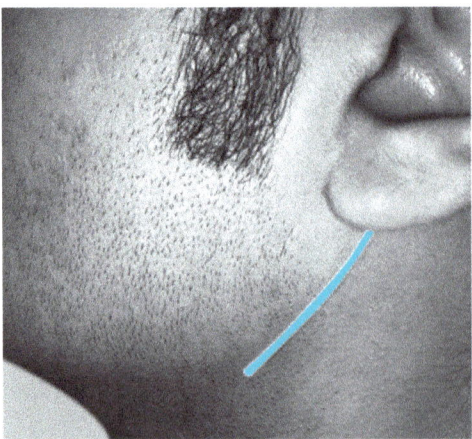

Fig. 8: Retromandibular approach

Rhytidectomy Approach (Fig. 9)

Major tumor resections may require more extensive joint exposure, and several authors have reported on the use of the rhytidectomy incision. The endaural incision is extended in a curvilinear fashion around the mastoid tip, with an S-shaped extension ending in a submandibular incision. This allows access to the entire posterior border of the mandible and allows for identification of the main trunk of the facial nerve.

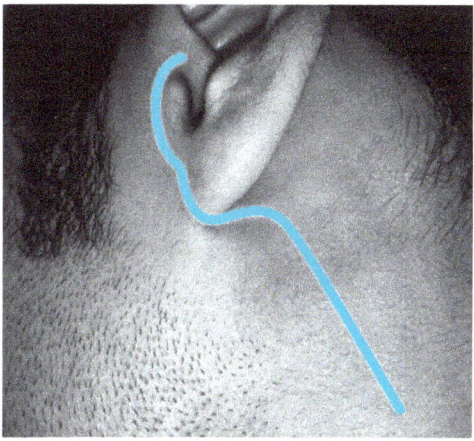

Fig. 9: Rhytidectomy approach

Trans-tragal Incision (Fig. 10)

The incision is a combination of the hockey-stick and endaural incisions. Its inferior part runs within the ear on the posterior face of the tragus; the tragal cartilage is transected together with the retrotragal skin and included in the anterior skin flap. This incision is commonly used for diacapitular condylar fractures.

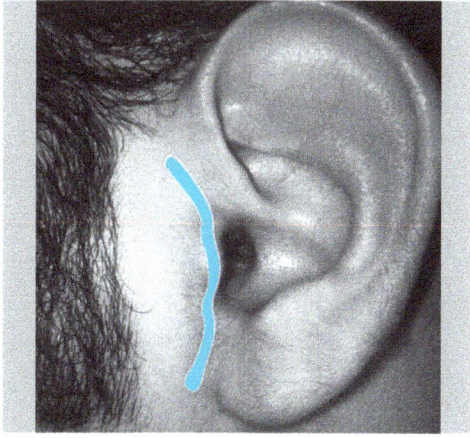

Fig. 10: Trans-tragal incision

Coronal Approach (Fig. 11)

Hemicoronal (unilateral incision) and bicoronal or coronal incision (bilateral incision) is more extensive, but versatile surgical approach to the upper and middle regions of the facial skeleton, including the zygomatic arch and the TM joint areas. It provides excellent access to these areas with minimum complications.

A major advantage is that most of the scar is hidden within the hairline, when the incision is extended into the preauricular area, the surgical scar is inconspicuous. This incision can be utilized for more extensive bilateral involvement.

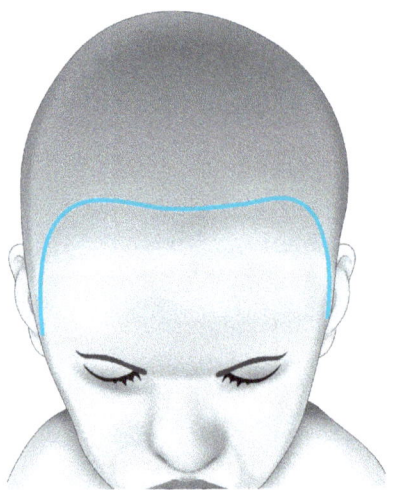

Fig. 11: Coronal approach

TMJ Capsular Incisions (Fig. 12)

Horizontal incision over the lateral rim of the glenoid fossa—The lateral ligament, capsule, and periosteum are reflected inferiorly en masse. Diskal or posterior attachment connections, or both, to the lateral capsule are dissected sharply with scissors to the level of the condylar neck.

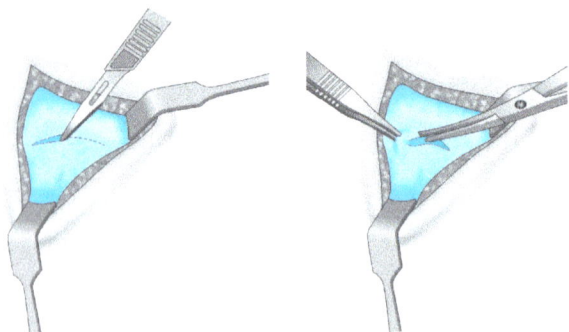

Fig. 12: TMJ capsular incisions

Horizontal incision below the lateral rim of the glenoid fossa—A no. 11 blade may be used to puncture into the superior joint space at the level of the lateral diskocapsular sulcus.

Horizontal incisions above and below the disk—The horizontal approach above and below the disk leaves some of the capsule and ligament attached to the disk or remodeled retrodiskal tissue.

L-shaped incision—A horizontal incision is made at or below the lateral rim of the glenoid fossa. The horizontal incision is then joined by either an anterior or posterior vertical extension. The posterior vertical incision carries the risk of severing the retrodiskal tissue. The anterior vertical incision should not be placed farther anteriorly than the tubercle to avoid injury to the facial nerve. The capsule and ligament are then reflected either anteroinferiorly or posteroinferiorly.

T-shaped incision—A horizontal incision is joined by a vertical incision to create a T-shaped incision over the midportion of the glenoid fossa.

Cross-hair incision—Dissection of the posterior attachment of the lateral ligament and capsule may be tedious with the cross-hair incision.

Open-sky incision—In the open-sky incision two horizontal incisions are joined by a central vertical incision.

Vertical incision—After a vertical incision is made, the capsular flaps are reflected anteriorly and posteriorly to expose the posterior attachment and disk.

CHAPTER

12

Flaps

Flap is a tissue may be soft tissue or hard tissue which is used to close the primary defect caused due to surgical ablation.

Flaps may be divided into local flaps and distant flaps. In this chapter, we shall see how to plan the incisions of these flaps.

LOCAL FLAPS

Forehead Flaps Incision (Fig. 1)

- **Lateral forehead flap (McGregor):** Based on superficial temporal artery vessels. It is used to close external defects of face, intraoral defects of buccal mucosa, cheek, etc.
- **Forehead scalping flap:** It is used for subtotal or total nasal reconstruction with partial reconstruction of the upper lip and cheek

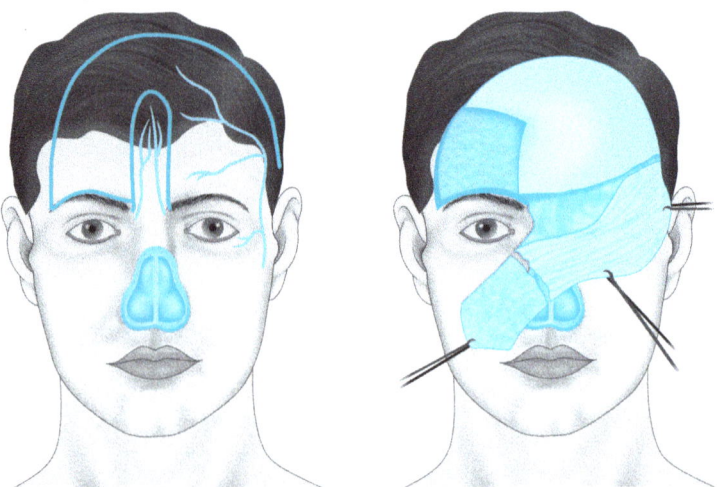

Fig. 1: Forehead flaps incision

- **Median forehead flap:** Based on supraorbital artery for defects of nose and supracialiary defects (Fig. 2).

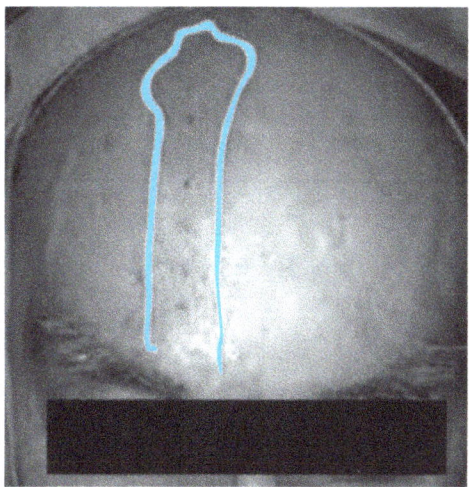

Fig. 2: Median forehead flap

Nasolabial Flap (Fig. 3)

The flap is soft, easily textured and has a convexity that matches well with that of the ala. This match is especially important. The nasolabial flap is designed so that the cheek scar is hidden within the nasolabial crease. Traditionally, the nasolabial flap has been used extensively for alar reconstruction and is viewed by many as the procedure of choice for this defect. The nasolabial flap is also commonly used in sidewall, columella, and intraoral reconstruction.

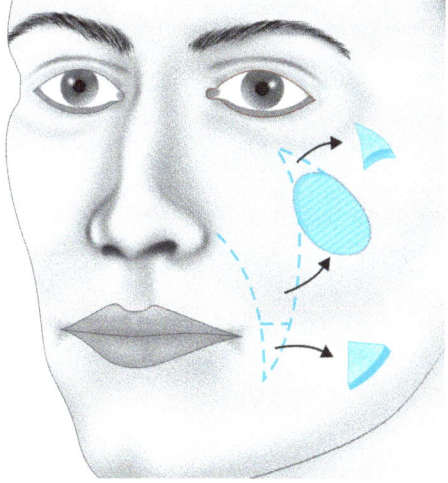

Fig. 3: Nasolabial flap

REGIONAL FLAPS

Pectoralis Major Myocutaneous Flap (Fig. 4)

The pectoralis major myocutaneous flap (PMMC) and myofascial flap variation are utilized in a large variety of head and neck reconstructive procedures that can include coverage of mucosal and/or cutaneous defects. The extent of coverage and the reach of the flap are dependent on the anatomy of the patient, modifications of the standard techniques of elevation, and inset. The upper limits are generally considered the zygomatic arch area externally and the superior tonsillar pole internally.

Landmarks

- Identify the clavicle, ipsilateral sternal border, xiphoid, and humeral insertion of the pectoralis muscle
- The course of the pectoral branch of the thoracoacromial artery can be identified by drawing a line from the xyphoid to the acromion. A second line perpendicular to this line is drawn that bisects the clavicle. The course of the artery corresponds to the line drawn from the midpoint of the clavicle continuing to the medial portion of the acromion to xyphoid line

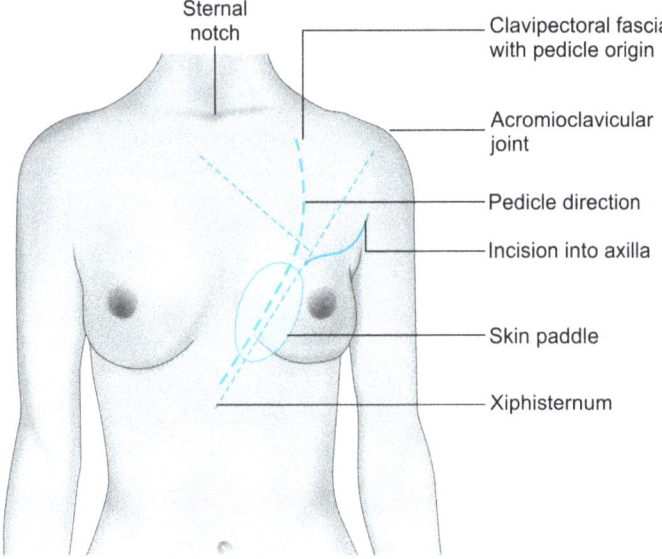

Fig. 4: Incision for PMMC Flap

Skin Paddle

- Size and location of skin paddle depends on reconstructive requirements. Standard skin paddle is located at the inferomedial border of the pectoralis major muscle that is inserting on the lateral border of the sternum and the 2nd to 6th costal cartilage

- Skin overlying any portion of the muscle may be utilized
- The larger the skin paddle harvested, the higher the likelihood the skin will survive the transfer due to the increased number of myocutaneous perforators
- For additional length, the skin paddle may be extended as a random-pattern flap beyond the inferior edge of the muscle belly
- Small flaps extended beyond the inferior muscle edge may exhibit an absence of myocutaneous perforators
- The myofascial flap is raised without a skin paddle.

Deltopectoral Flap (Fig. 5)

The deltopectoral (DP) flap, also called by some as the Bakamjian flap, was actually first described by Aymard in 1917. All flaps were harvested as fasciocutaneous flaps based on second and third perforators of the internal mammary artery arising from the deltopectoral groove. The skin medial to the DP groove is reliably nourished by the internal perforators, but the skin lateral to the DP groove is usually nourished by musculocutaneous perforators arising from the deltoid muscles. The extended portion of DP flap beyond the DP groove is therefore, essentially a random pattern flap. Whenever this is necessary, we limit our extension within the 1:1 base-to-length ratio.

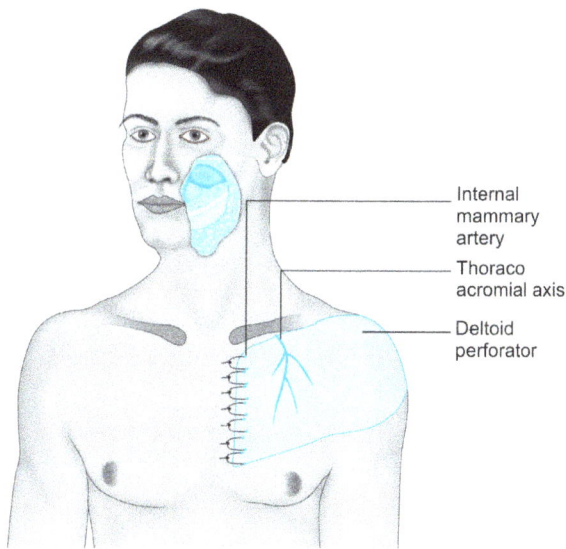

Fig. 5: Deltopectoral flap

Fibula Flap

The fibula free flap provides a long, strong segment of bone for use in reconstructive surgery. It can be harvested as a purely osseous flap or can include a large fasciocutaneous component if needed. The pedicle runs the length of the fibula, with perforators extending to supply the skin paddle. To date, no other flap is capable of providing such a long segment of bone; up to

26 cm can be taken without affecting leg function. A segment of bone must be preserved distally, however, to support the ankle, and proximally to avoid injury to the peroneal nerve.

Incision for Fibula Flap (Fig. 6)

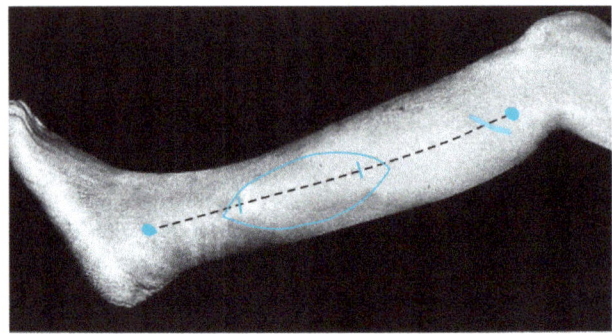

Fig. 6: Incision for fibula flap

Iliac Flap

The deep circumflex iliac artery (DCIA) bone flap provides a large concave segment of bone suitable for reconstruction of the upper extremity, lower extremity and mandible. Although the fibula has often replaced the DCIA when bone reconstruction is necessary, especially in the mandible, the DCIA provides a large segment of cancellous bone up to 15 cm long and 6 cm wide. The fibula, in contrast, supplies only cortical bone. In addition, when the peroneal artery inflow is not adequate, or the lower extremities have been injured, the DCIA is an excellent choice when a large block of bone is necessary in lieu of the fibula.

Incision for Iliac Flap (Fig. 7)

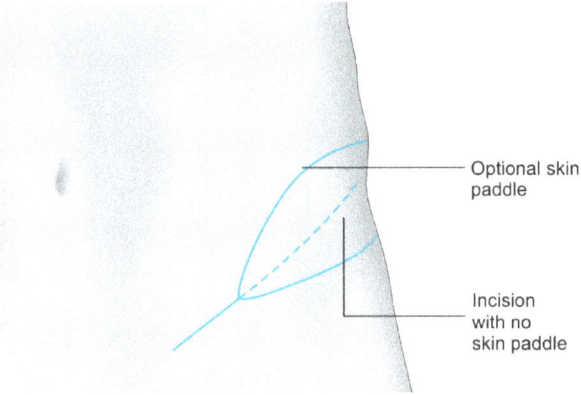

Fig. 7: The incision is marked just superior to the inguinal ligament. A skin paddle is optional

Anterolateral Thigh Flap

The axis of the surface of the septum between the rectus femoris and the vastus lateralis is marked by a line connecting the anterior superior iliac spine and the lateral patella. This line is divided into thirds for purposes of outlining the flap. The junction of the proximal and middle third is often the site of a perforator that pierces the tensor fascia lata. This point can be incorporated in the flap to keep the TFL perforator as a "lifeboat" in the rare circumstance when the distal perforators are of poor quality or injured during dissection. The junction of the middle and distal third is marked and is also incorporated into the flap. The flap design can be adjusted depending on findings of a Doppler exam.

Incision of ALT Flap (Figs 8A and B)

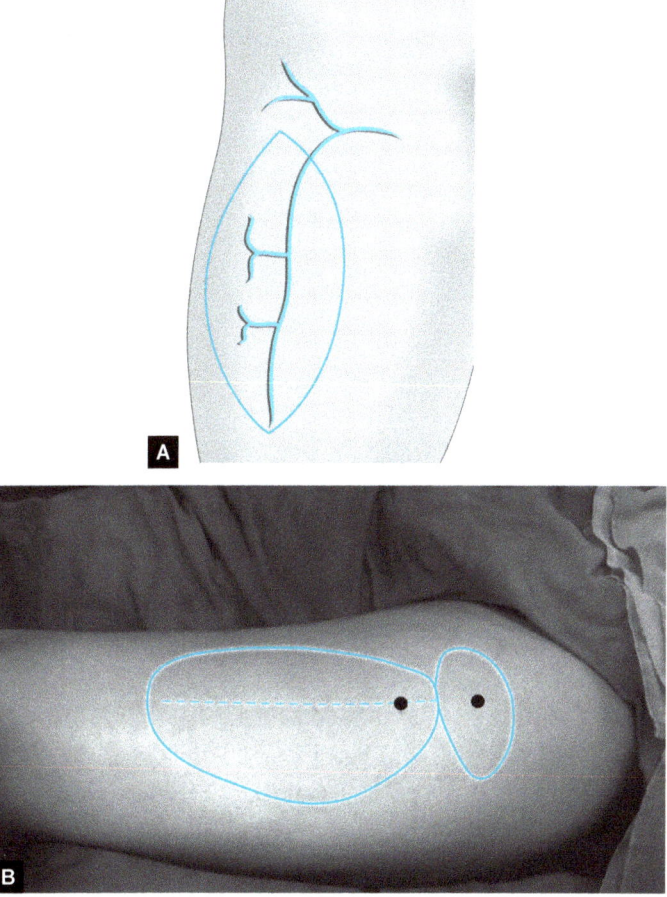

Figs 8A and B: Incision of ALT flap

Scapular Flap

The scapula flap has been used extensively for oromandibular and oromaxillary reconstruction. The ability to three-dimensionally orient the bone with respect to the skin paddle has made it a popular flap choice in central facial, orbital, and maxillary reconstruction.

Incision of Scapular Flap (Fig. 9)

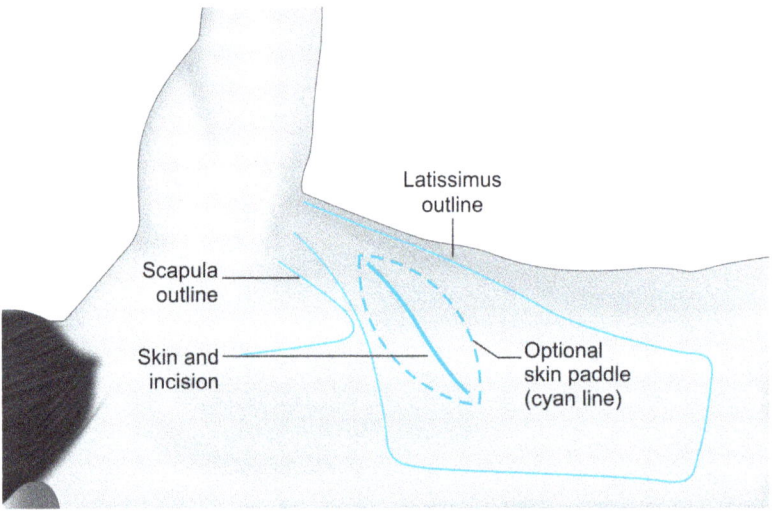

Fig. 9: Incision of scapular flap

Radial Forearm Flap (Fig. 10)

Radial forearm flap is the work horse for tongue defects. Its is based on radial artery and vein. Cephalic vein can also be taken due to its greater width and caliber for microvascular anastomosis.

The incision is usually placed on ulnar side with a distance of 1 cm from the wrist. The vertical incision is placed at the junction of brachioradialis and flexor carpi muscle.

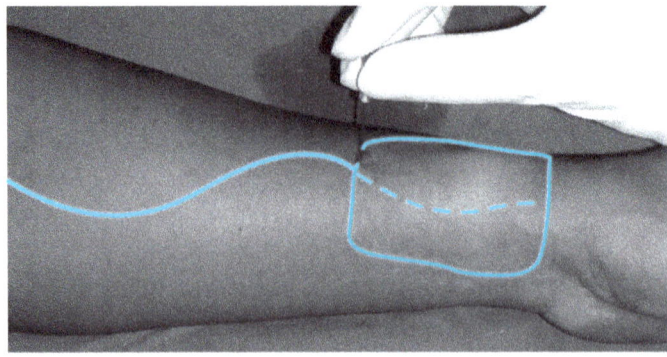

Fig. 10: Radial forearm flap

LIP RECONSTRUCTION FLAPS

Lip Shave (Figs 11A to D)

Given along the mucosa and mucocutaneous junction.

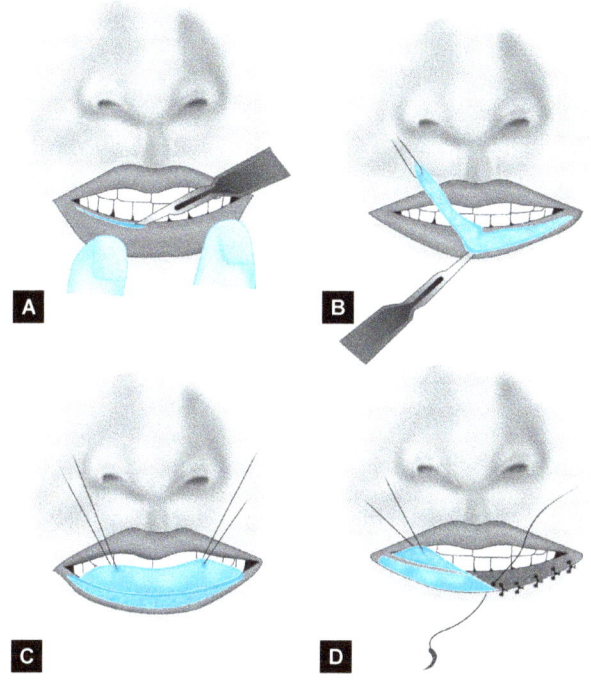

Figs 11A to D: Lip shave

Buccal Mucosal Advancement Flap

Relaxing incision on mucosa at deep buccal sulcus. Mucosa elevated deep to salivary glands and superficial to orbicularis oris muscle (Figs 12A to C).

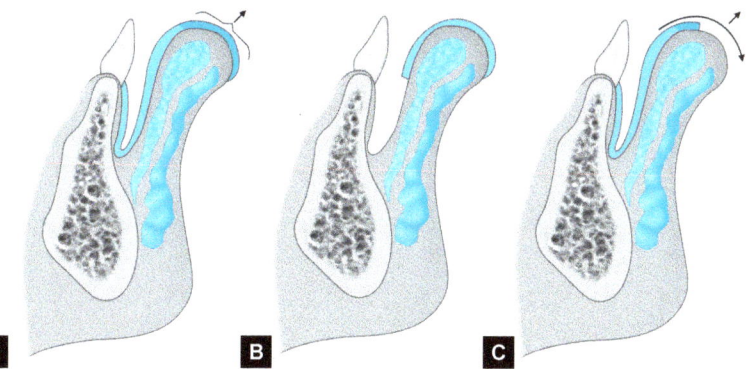

Figs 12A to C: Buccal mucosal advancement flap

V or W Wedge Resection

Most common incision for less than 1/3rd defects of lip (Figs 13A to F).

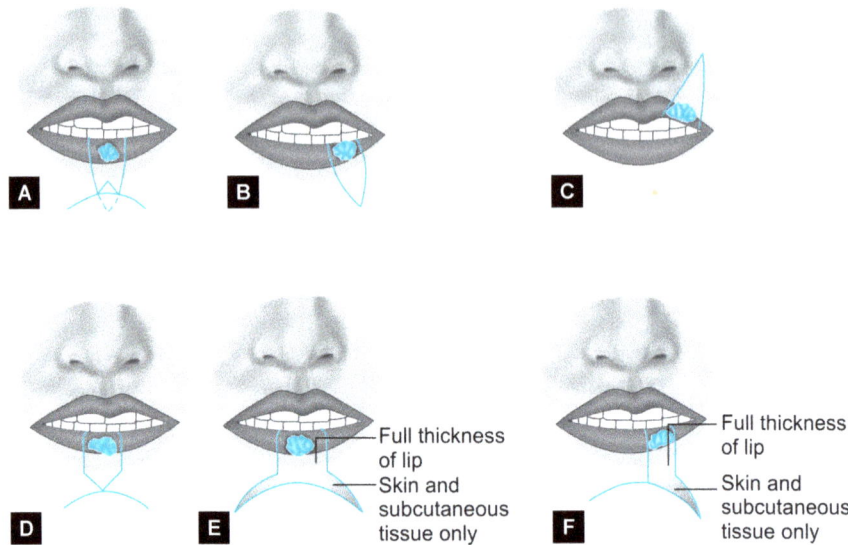

Figs 13A to F: V or W wedge resection

Lower Lip Rectangular Flaps

Incision for more than 2/3rds defects of lip (Figs 14A and B).

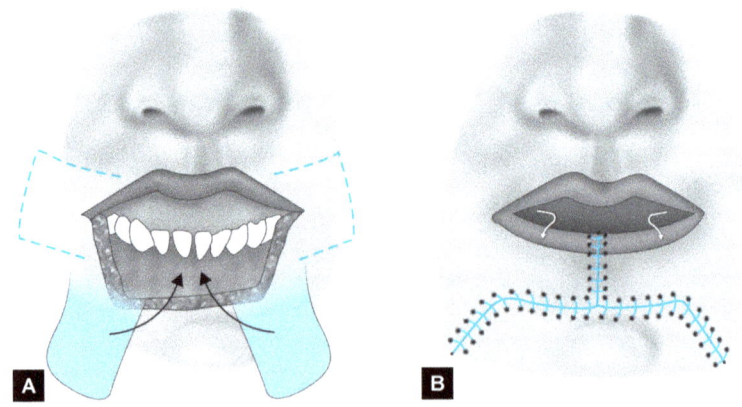

Figs 14A and B: Lower lip rectangular flaps

Step Ladder Method (Fig. 15)

- Horizontal component of step excisions—1/2 width of defect
- Vertical dimension 8–10 mm, 2 to 4 steps are made. This can be used to close defects up to 2/3rds of lip length.

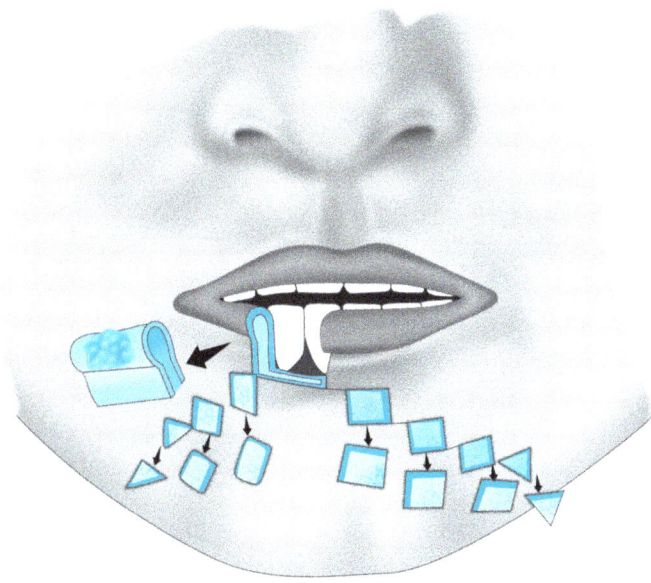

Fig. 15: Step ladder method

Abbe Flap (Figs 16A to D)

- Junction of middle and lateral 1/3rd of upper lip
- Away from philtral columns and commissure
- Maximum flap size—2–3 cm.

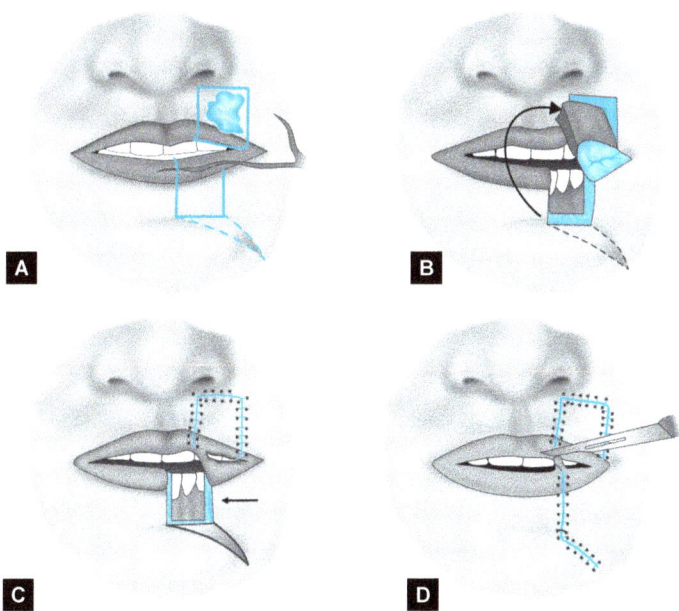

Figs 16A to D: Abbe flap

Bilateral Extraphiltral Cross-lip Flaps

Less than 1/3rd defects of lip (Figs 17A and B).

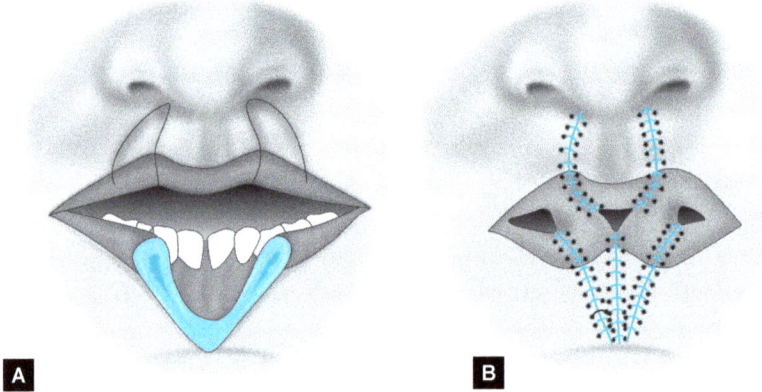

Figs 17A and B: Bilateral extraphiltral cross-lip flaps

Abbe Estlander Flap (Figs 18A to C)

Incision for 1/3rd to 2/3rd defects of lip.

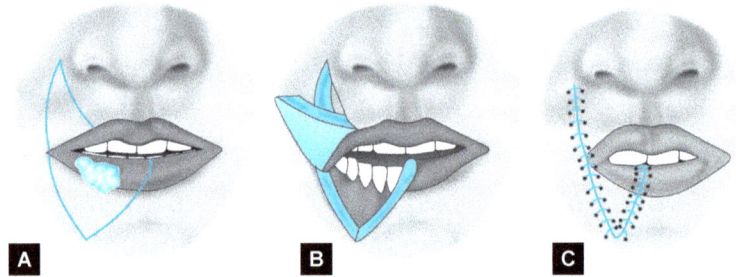

Figs 18A to C: Abbe estlander flap

Gillies Fan Flap

Incision for more than 2/3rd defects of lip (Fig. 19A to C).

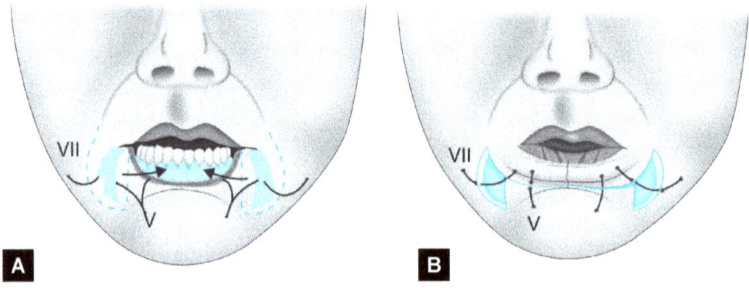

Figs 19A to C: *Contd...*

Flaps | 71

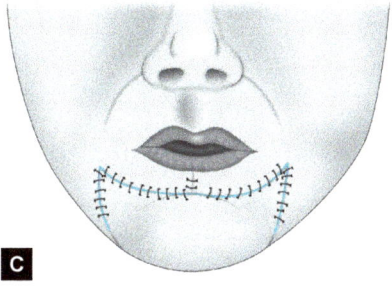

Figs 19A to C: Gillies fan flap

Bernard Burow's Procedure

Incision for more than 2/3rd defects of lip (Figs 20A and B).

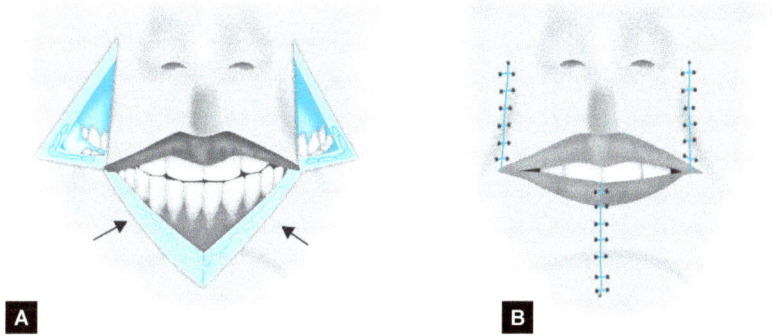

Figs 20A and B: Bernard burow's procedure

Perialar Crescentic Skin Excisions

Incision for more than 2/3rd defects of lip (Figs 21A and B).

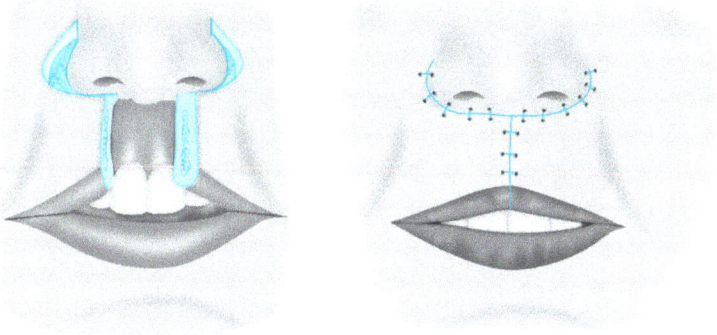

Figs 21A and B: Perialar crescentic skin excisions

CHEEK RECONSTRUCTION

- Aesthetic units (Fig. 22)
  - Zone I
    ◊ Suborbital.
  - Zone II
    ◊ Preauricular.
  - Zone III
    ◊ Buccomandibular
    ◊ Includes oral lining in full thickness defects.

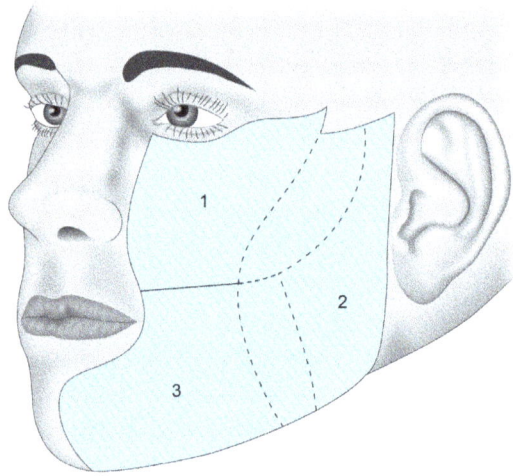

Fig. 22: Cheek reconstruction: Aesthetic units

ZONE 1

Cervicofacial Flap (Fig. 23)

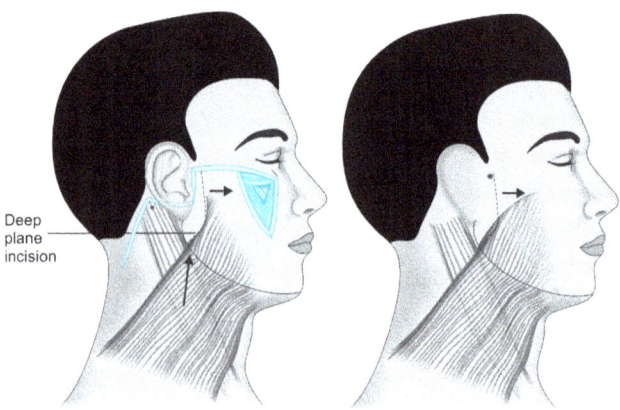

Fig. 23: Cervicofacial flap

ZONE II and III

Cervicopectoral Flap (Fig. 24)

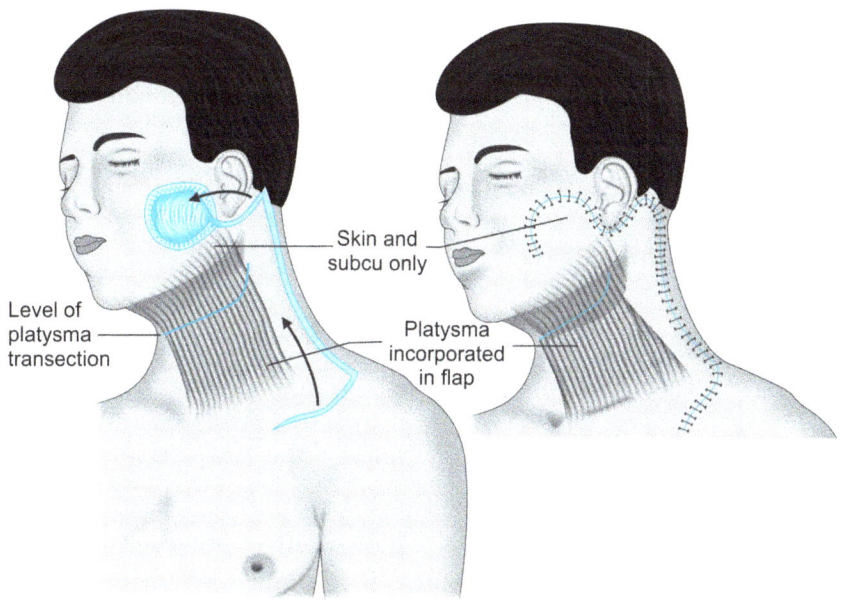

Fig. 24: Cervicopectoral flap

CHAPTER
13

Aesthetic Surgery

RHINOPLASTY

Incision and Approaches (Fig. 1)

There are two most common approaches to perform rhinoplasty. The first one is a closed (endonasal) technique and the other one is an open (external) technique.

In reconstructive rhinoplasty, the open technique is used. This provides excellent exposure of the nasal anatomy and allows for a more precise rhinoplasty. This requires a very small incision along the thinnest part of the skin (columella) between the nostrils. The incision which is only 3–4 mm long normally heals without any visible scar.

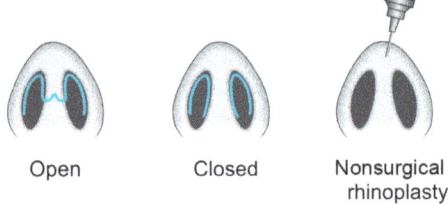

Fig. 1: Open vs closed rhinoplasty

Incisions Types

Types of incisions are as follows:
- Trans-columellar
- Transfixion
- Hemitransfixion
- Infracartilage (marginal)
- Intercartilage
- Cartilage-splitting.

Aesthetic Surgery | 75

Trans-Columellar Incision (Fig. 2)

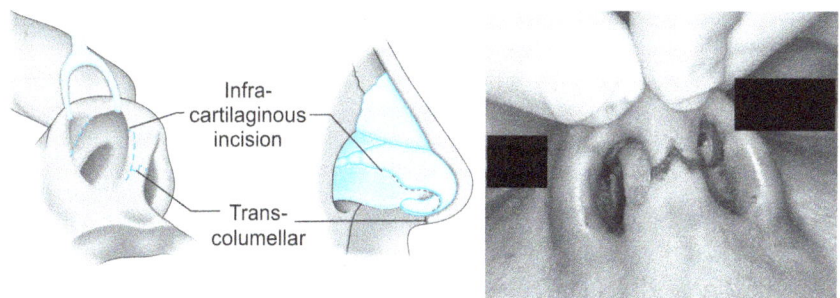

Fig. 2: Trans-columellar incision

Transfixion Incision (Fig. 3)

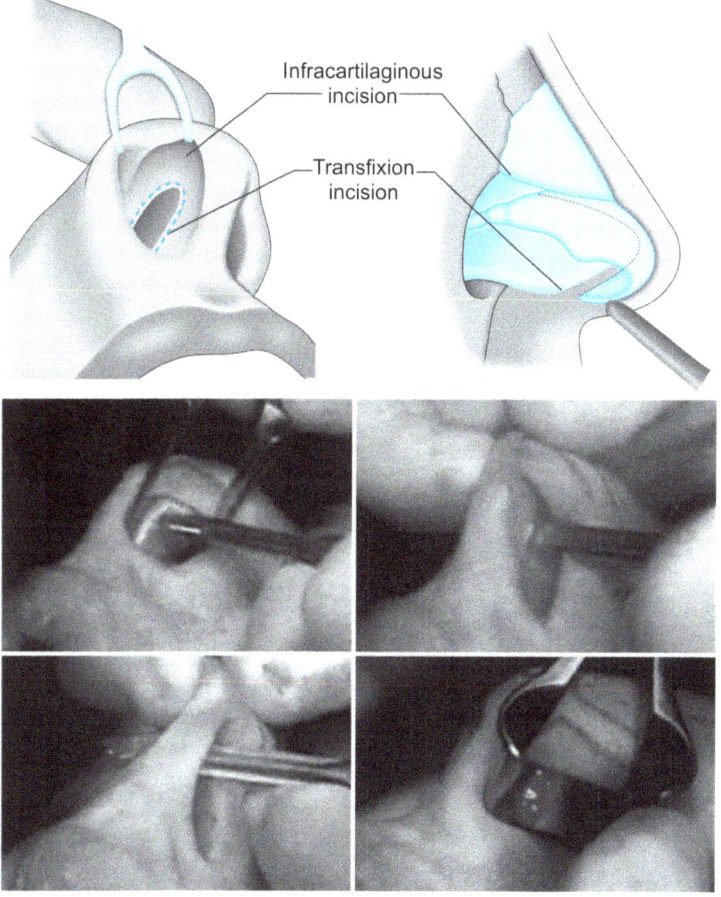

Fig. 3: Transfixion incision

Infracartilage (Marginal) Incision (Fig. 4)

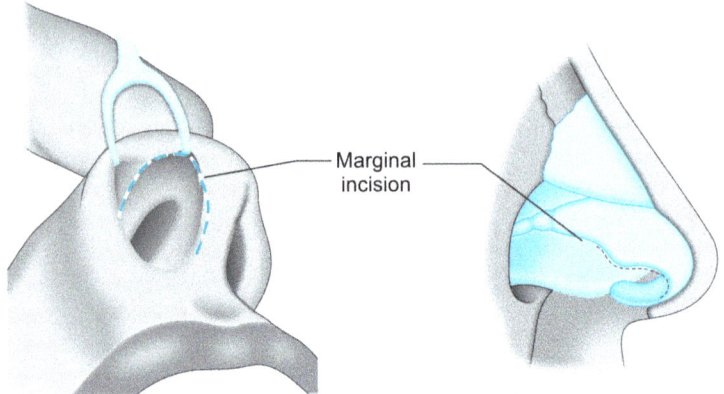

Fig. 4: Infracartilage (Marginal) incision

INTERCARTILAGINOUS and CARTILAGE SPLITTING INCISION (Fig. 5)

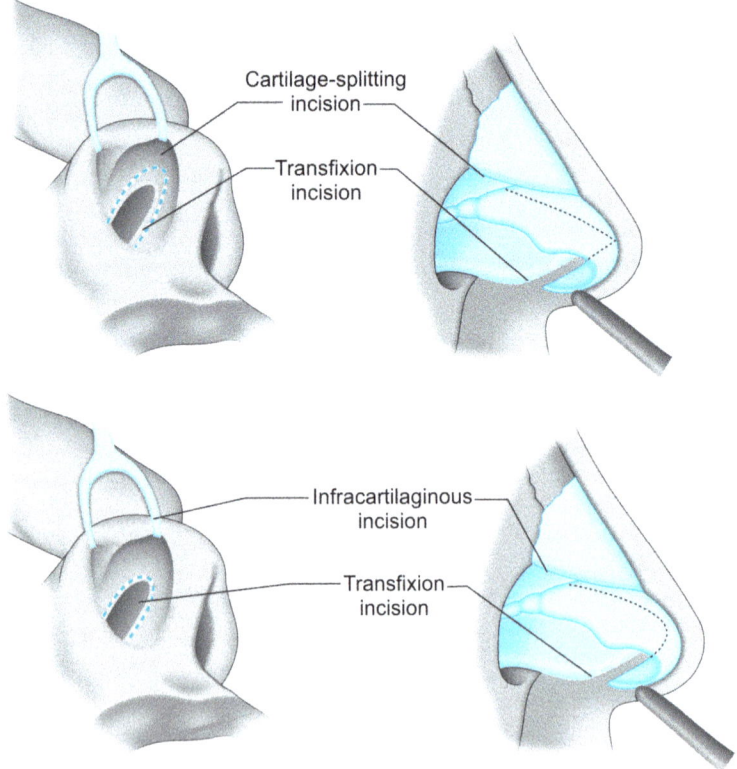

Fig. 5: Intercartilaginous and cartilage splitting incision

Brow Lift Procedures (Fig. 6)

Mark the shape and position of the eyebrows. It is important to examine which part of the eyebrow needs to be raised the most and which needs to be raised the least. The point in the eyebrow that is to be raised the most is transferred vertically up to the hairline.

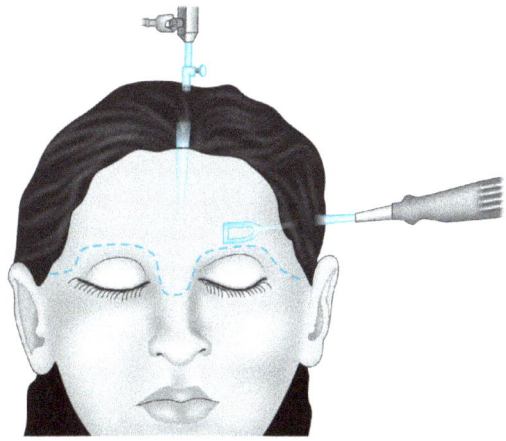

Fig. 6: Brow lift procedures

Make an incision at the front edge of the hairline along the midline, followed by two vertical incisions on each side, which correspond to the marked point of each eyebrow. If the patient has an abnormally high or receding hairline, these incisions can be made in nonhair-bearing skin provided that intradermal sutures are used upon completion. Hereafter, you begin dissection from the central incision and release the periosteum blindly but without destroying it.

Other Incisions (Fig. 7)

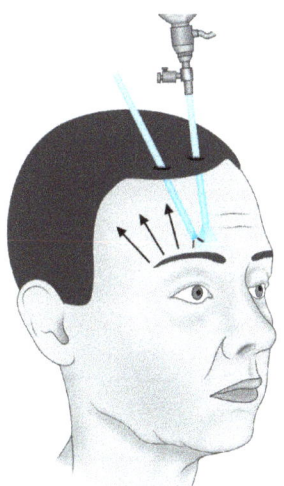

Fig. 7: Other incisions

LIP AUGMENTATION

Types of incisions are shown in Figure 8:

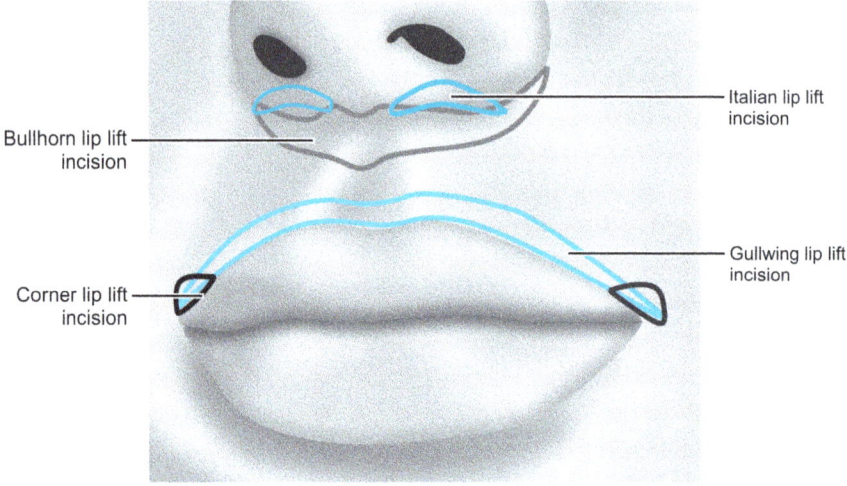

Fig. 8: Lip augmentation

Bibliography

1. Ellis E, Zide MF (eds). Surgical approaches to the facial skeleton. Lippincott Williams & Wilkins; 2006.
2. Fonseca RJ, et al. Oral and maxillofacial trauma. Elsevier Health Sciences: 2013.
3. Hupp, James R, and Myron R. Tucker, eds. Contemporary oral and maxillofacial surgery, 3rd ed. St Louis, Mosby; 1998.
4. Malik NA. Textbook of oral and maxillofacial surgery. Jaypee Brothers Medical Publishers: 2008.
5. Miloro M, et al. Peterson's principles of oral and maxillofacial surgery. Vol. 1. PMPH-USA; 2004.
6. Perrott DH. "Textbook of Oral & Maxillofacial Surgery."
7. Spiessl B (ed). New concepts in maxillofacial bone surgery. Springer Science & Business Media; 2012.
8. Textbook of Face and Reconstruction, Mcgregor.
9. Text book of Oral & maxillofacial Surgery, Peter Wardbooth.

Index

Page numbers followed by *f* refer to figure

A

Abbe Estlander flap 69, 69*f*, 70, 70*f*
Aesthetic surgery 74
Al-Kayat and Bramley's incision 51
Apron incision 33*f*
  modified 33*f*
Auricle 6
Axillary incision 42

B

Bardach palatoplasty 49, 49*f*
Basic preauricular incision,
        modifications of 52
Berke lateral canthotomy incision,
        modified 18, 19*f*
Bernard Burow's procedure 71, 71*f*
Bicoronal scalp incision 32f
Blair's incision 51
  modified 39, 40
Blepharoplasty, lower 18
Boomerang incision 33*f*, 34, 35*f*
  bilateral 33*f*
Borle's extention 28
Bowerman's incision 21
Brow
  incision, lateral 15, 16*f*
  lift procedures 77, 77*f*
Buccal mucosal advancement
        flap 67, 67*f*
Burbosa incision 31

C

Canthotomy incision, lateral 19
Carotid body tumor incision line 43*f*
Cartilage splitting incision 76
Cephalic vein 66
Cervicofacial flap 72, 72*f*
Cervicopectoral flap 73, 73*f*
Cheek
  incisions 31
  reconstruction 72, 72*f*

Cleft
  lip 44
    incisions 44
  palate 49
Commissures 6
  split 30, 30*f*
Conley incision 37, 37*f*
Coronal incision 17, 19
Cranial nerve 2
Crokett's incision 31
Cross-hair incision 59

D

Da-Vinci robotic system 41
Deep circumflex iliac artery 64
Deltopectoral flap 63, 63*f*
Dingman's incision 21, 22*f*, 51

E

Endaural incision 51
Envelope incision 12, 12*f*, 13, 15
Extraphiltral cross-lip flaps,
        bilateral 70, 70*f*
Eye incision 28
Eyelids 6

F

Face, fourth dimension of 1
Facelift incision 40, 40*f*
Facial nerve 2
  branches 54
Fibula flap 63, 64, 64*f*
Forehead
  flaps 60
    incision 60, 60*f*
    scalping flap 60
Frontal bone fractures 19
Frontoethmoidal lynch incision 18, 19*f*
Furlow Z-plasty 49, 49*f*

G

George Crile incision 35, 36f
Gillies fan flap 70, 71f
Gillies principles 9
Glenoid fossa 58, 59
Gluck-Sorenson incision 42f

H

Hayter incision 30, 30f
Hetter's incision 38, 38f
Hockey incision, bilateral 36, 37f
Hockey stick incision 34, 34f
Horizontal radix incision 23f

I

Iliac flap 64, 64
Incision 38, 38f, 39, 46, 48f, 51, 64, 77, 77f
   concepts of 6
   principles of 2
   types 74, 78
Infracartilage incision 76, 76f
Infraorbital incision 15, 17f
Infratemporal fossa 32
Intercartilaginous and cartilage splitting incision 76f
Internal jugular vein 34
Intraoral incision 14, 15f, 17, 40, 51

J

Jaegar Jugal incision 31

L

Laryngeal tumors 42
Lempert's endaural approach, modifications of 54
Lid percutaneous incision, lower 19
Lip
   augmentation 78, 78f
   reconstruction flaps 67
   rectangular flaps, lower 68, 68f
   shave 67, 67f
   split incision, modified 30, 31f
L-shaped incision 11, 11f, 59
Lymph node excisions 43
Lymphadenectomy 32, 33f

M

Mandibular fractures 13
Marginal incision 76, 76f
Maxillary
   buccal sulcus approach 17
   fractures 15, 16
   neoplasms 26
Maxillectomy 28f
Maxillofacial fractures 13
McFee incision 35, 35f
McGregor incision 29, 29f
Median forehead flap 61, 61f
Midface degloving incision 28
Milliard rotation 44, 45, 45f
Mini-parotid incision 39, 39f
Mucoperiosteal flaps 49f

N

Nasal
   alae 6
   tip 6
Nasolabial flap 61, 61f
Naso-orbito-ethmoid fractures 20
Neck
   dissections 32
   incision 31
   swellings, lateral 43
Necklace incision 41f
Non-lymphatic structures 34

O

Open sky incision 59
Oral cavity neoplasms 28
Orbit fractures 18, 18f
Orbital
   incisions 19f
   rim, inferior 18

P

Paranasal sinus tumors, removal of 26
Pectoralis major myocutaneous flap 62
Perialar crescentic skin excisions 71, 71f
Postauricular incision 51
Preauricular incision
   modifications of 53f
   parts of 52f

R

Radial forearm flap 66, 66*f*
Radical neck dissection 34
   modified 34
Reconstruction, principles of 9
Relaxed skin-tension lines 6
Retroauricular incision 40, 40*f*
Retromandibular incision 13, 14*f*
Rhinoplasty 74
   open vs closed 74*f*
Rhinotomy 27
Rhytidectomy incision 51
Risdon's approach 134, 51, 55
Robson's incision 29, 29*f*
Roux-Trotter incision 29, 29*f*

S

Salivary gland neoplasm 39
Scapular flap 66
   incision of 66, 66*f*
Schobinger incision, modified 36, 36*f*
Seagul incision 21, 22*f*
Skin
   incision 54
      lower limit of 54
   paddle 62
Spinal accessory nerve 34
Stallard-Wright lateral orbitotomy
        incision 18, 19*f*
Step ladder method 68, 69*f*
Sternocleidomastoid 34
   muscle, posterior border of 34
Submandibular incision 31, 40
Superficial temporal artery 54
Supraciliary incision 20
Supraomohyoid neck dissection 33, 33*f*
Surgical scalpel blades, types of 3

T

Temporomandibular joint 51
   capsular incisions 58, 58*f*
Tennison-Randall flap 46, 46*f*
Thigh flap 65
Thoma's incision 51
Thyroid tumors 40
Traditional parotidectomy incision 39
Transaxillary thyroidectomy 41, 42*f*
Transcaruncular incision 18, 19*f*, 22, 75
Trans-columellar incision 75*f*
Transconjunctival
   lower lid incision 19
   medial orbitotomy 19
Transfixion incision 75, 75*f*
Trans-tragal incision 51, 57, 57*f*

V

V or W wedge resection 68*f*
Vermilion 6
Vertical incision 20, 20*f*, 59
Vestibular incision 14, 15, 15*f*, 16*f*
Visor incision 31, 31*f*
von Langenbeck incision 29, 29*f*
von Langenbeck palatoplasty 50, 50*f*

W

Ward's incision 10, 10*f*
   modified 10, 11*f*
Weber-Ferguson incision 27, 27*f*

Z

Z-shaped incision 28
Zygomatic arch 58
Zygomatic complex fractures 15

www.ingramcontent.com/pod-product-compliance
Lightning Source LLC
Chambersburg PA
CBHW040517220526
45473CB00012B/2895